Contents

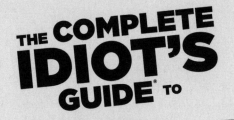

Low-Carb Meals

Second Edition

by Lucy Beale and Sandy G. Couvillon, MS, LDN, RD

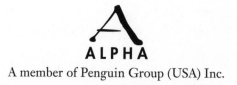

A member of Penguin Group (USA) Inc.

y: To my mother, Ann Murphy Rusnock

Sandy: To my three favorite food tasters: Brian, Courtney, and Brad

ALPHA BOOKS

Published by Penguin Group (USA) Inc.

Penguin Group (USA) Inc., 375 Hudson Street, New York, New York 10014, USA • Penguin Group (Canada), 90 Eglinton Avenue East, Suite 700, Toronto, Ontario M4P 2Y3, Canada (a division of Pearson Penguin Canada Inc.) • Penguin Books Ltd., 80 Strand, London WC2R 0RL, England • Penguin Ireland, 25 St. Stephen's Green, Dublin 2, Ireland (a division of Penguin Books Ltd.) • Penguin Group (Australia), 250 Camberwell Road, Camberwell, Victoria 3124, Australia (a division of Pearson Australia Group Pty. Ltd.) • Penguin Books India Pvt. Ltd., 11 Community Centre, Panchsheel Park, New Delhi—110 017, India • Penguin Group (NZ), 67 Apollo Drive, Rosedale, North Shore, Auckland 1311, New Zealand (a division of Pearson New Zealand Ltd.) • Penguin Books (South Africa) (Pty.) Ltd., 24 Sturdee Avenue, Rosebank, Johannesburg 2196, South Africa • Penguin Books Ltd., Registered Offices: 80 Strand, London WC2R 0RL, England

Copyright © 2012 by Lucy Beale and Sandy G. Couvillon

International Standard Book Number: 978-1-61564-196-3
Library of Congress Catalog Card Number: 2011943396

19   18   17   15   14   13   12   11   10   9

Interpretation of the printing code: The rightmost number of the first series of numbers is the year of the book's printing; the rightmost number of the second series of numbers is the number of the book's printing. For example, a printing code of 12-1 shows that the first printing occurred in 2012.

Printed in the United States of America

Note: This publication contains the opinions and ideas of its author. It is intended to provide helpful and informative material on the subject matter covered. It is sold with the understanding that the authors and publisher are not engaged in rendering professional services in the book. If the reader requires personal assistance or advice, a competent professional should be consulted.

The authors and publisher specifically disclaim any responsibility for any liability, loss, or risk, personal or otherwise, which is incurred as a consequence, directly or indirectly, of the use and application of any of the contents of this book.

Most Alpha books are available at special quantity discounts for bulk purchases for sales promotions, premiums, fund-raising, or educational use. Special books, or book excerpts, can also be created to fit specific needs. For details, write: Special Markets, Alpha Books, 375 Hudson Street, New York, NY 10014.

Publisher: *Marie Butler-Knight*
Associate Publisher: *Mike Sanders*
Executive Managing Editor: *Billy Fields*
Senior Acquisitions Editor: *Tom Stevens*
Development Editor: *Nancy D. Lewis*
Senior Production Editor: *Janette Lynn*

Copy Editor: *Cate Schwenk*
Cover Designer: *William Thomas*
Book Designers: *William Thomas/Rebecca Batchelor*
Indexer: *Brad Herriman*
Layout: *Ayanna Lacey*
Senior Proofreader: *Laura Caddell*

Appendix

Introduction

There's a certain rhythm to cooking and eating low carb. Once you get into the flow of it, you'll be cooking low carb with joy and delight for the rest of your life.

In this book, you'll find mouthwatering recipes for all your daily meals and special occasions. You'll be able to use regular grocery store ingredients to make scrumptious main courses, side dishes, and, yes, even desserts, breads, and chocolate goodies. You can eat them with confidence, knowing that you are eating healthfully, managing your weight, and maintaining your overall well-being.

How This Book Is Organized

This book is divided into six parts:

Part 1, The Low-Carb Way of Eating, gives you an overview of low-carb eating and cooking. You'll learn which carbs count and which don't, how to use the glycemic index (GI), and how to eat a balanced low-carb diet. You'll learn to create a positive mind-set while eating delicious foods in the best portion sizes.

Part 2, Breakfasts and Lunches, gives you great recipes for both quick and leisurely breakfasts. You'll learn how to make low-carb breakfasts in advance so you can eat on the run. And you'll learn low-carb recipes for packed lunches as well as the kind you eat at home.

Part 3, Main Dish Entrées, contains recipes for your main meat or fish course. These include yummy beef, pork, poultry, seafood, and fish dishes. You'll use these recipes for dinner and also for lunches and even breakfast.

Part 4, Main Dish Combinations, gives you recipes for one-pot meals, soups, stews, eggs, cheese, and main-dish salads. "One pot" is the new term for casseroles. With these recipes, you'll have plenty of variety for interesting eating. Many of them contain added vegetables and fruits.

Part 5, Side Dishes, provides you with recipes for snacks and appetizers for those times when you really need to have a little something to tide you over until the next meal. You'll find recipe chapters for vegetable, fruit, and salad side dishes.

Part 6, Extras: Treats and Starches, is filled with the comfort foods we all enjoy. You'll find recipes for breads, grains, and potatoes. And if you have a sweet tooth, you'll enjoy our great collection of luscious dessert recipes, plus a whole chapter on chocolate.

Tasty Bites

The sidebars in this book offer low-carb notes and tips, recipe ideas, cooking cautions, and definitions. Here's what to look for:

TABLE TALK

These sidebars give good information and notes on cooking and eating low-carb foods.

DEFINITION

The definitions of words and concepts in these sidebars increase your knowledge of low-carb eating and cooking.

HOT POTATO

Watch out! These sidebars help you avoid errors in cooking procedures and things that may hamper your low-carb eating plan.

RECIPE FOR SUCCESS

Use these sidebars on how to serve and enjoy each recipe to increase your dining pleasure.

But Wait! There's More!

Have you logged on to idiotsguides.com lately? If you haven't, go there now! As a bonus to the book, we've included tons of additional low-carb information that you'll want to check out, all online. Point your browser to idiotsguides.com/lowcarbmeals, and enjoy!

Acknowledgments

Just as a good recipe tastes best when made with the finest ingredients, a cookbook succeeds best when given helpful and loving support.

Lucy Beale gives loving thanks to her husband, Patrick Partridge, for his caring interest and editing suggestions; to her late mother, Ann Murphy Rusnock, for years ago teaching her how to compose and create recipes; and to her co-author, Sandy Couvillon, for her steadfast work and commitment. The following people gave generously of their time and knowledge. Thanks to Rick Mendosa, Lori Beecher, Caryll Cram, Steve Burns, Margarita Guerra, Greg Terrell, Judy Webb, and Greg Davis. Lucy also thanks her newsletter readers and workshop participants who urged her to write a low-carb cookbook for them.

Lucy and Sandy thank Marilyn Allen, Bob DiForio, Coleen O'Shea, and Renee Wilmeth for their guidance in bringing this cookbook into reality.

Sandy Couvillon gives heartfelt thanks to her husband, Brian, for his support and understanding for the many evenings and weekends spent typing and calculating recipes. Much love to Brian and their children, Courtney and Brad, for helping her enjoy years of experimenting with recipes to find healthier and more delicious ways to combine ingredients. Thankfully she had many years of delectable recipes to fall back on from two loving, experienced cooks, her mom, Velma, and her mother-in-law, Stella. Two important family members cannot be left out as they have always been there to lend encouragement, her dad, Jim, and her brother, Jim. Many thanks to her co-author, Lucy, for her enthusiasm and energy that is reflected in this project.

Sincere gratitude and thanks go to her co-workers, who eagerly tasted and honestly rated many recipes for the book. Thanks to her clients who gave input into the types of recipes they needed to make low-carb eating fun. Sandy sends love and hugs to her many friends who supported this endeavor and understood when deadlines had to take first place. Without this love and support of family and friends this project could not have happened nor would it have been such fun.

Special Thanks to the Technical Reviewer

The Complete Idiot's Guide to Low-Carb Meals, Second Edition, was reviewed by an expert who double-checked the accuracy of what you'll learn here, to help us ensure that this book gives you everything you need to know about preparing low-carb meals. Special thanks are extended to Rhonda Lerner.

Trademarks

All terms mentioned in this book that are known to be or are suspected of being trademarks or service marks have been appropriately capitalized. Alpha Books and Penguin Group (USA) Inc. cannot attest to the accuracy of this information. Use of a term in this book should not be regarded as affecting the validity of any trademark or service mark.

The Low-Carb Way of Eating

Low-carb eating is here to stay. It works. It works for you and it makes you feel good—physically, mentally, and emotionally. Low-carb cooking is becoming not just a weight-loss or wellness remedy, but an art form.

The challenge with low-carb cooking is to cook up the most delicious foods with the right amount of carbohydrates—enough to satisfy your palate and your tastes, but not so many that you exceed your daily carb allotment. An additional challenge is to make every carbohydrate nutritionally beneficial for your best health, ideal weight, and overall well-being.

Fabulous low-carb cooking eliminates feelings of deprivation and, instead, makes you glad that your foods are satisfying and pleasurable.

Delicious Low-Carb Cooking

In This Chapter

- Low-carb eating is anything but boring
- Accommodating your daily carb allotment
- Counting carbs and the glycemic index

By the time you purchase this book, you've been on a quest. You're committed to eating low carb. You've been told or done enough research to know that this dietary plan is good for what seems to be ailing you. People choose low-carb eating as a solution to weight loss, diabetes, high blood pressure, heart conditions, autoimmune diseases, depression, and anxiety. You'll find as you eat low carb that it really works to help you achieve your health and wellness goals.

However, the dietary limitations of low-carb eating can seem to get very boring very fast. Fortunately, boring eating is not a requirement for eating low carb. Just the opposite can be true. In fact, the opposite needs to be true for a person to eat low carb day in and day out over years, in fact, over a lifetime.

As members of the human species, we are programmed biologically to seek out delicious and interesting foods. The good news is, you've found an entire cookbook that can satisfy your quest for scrumptious low-carb foods. In this chapter we define the parameters of counting carbs and show you how to use the glycemic index, which will help you learn how to make great selections when planning meals. And the recipes throughout the chapters definitely keep you from experiencing food boredom.

The Carb Count Limit

What constitutes low-carb eating varies with the experts. What we know is that you have to eat some carbs to stay happy and healthy. But the answer to how many isn't clear. The range of acceptable daily amounts swings from 15 to 250, depending on the expert.

Dr. Atkins, who led the movement to eating virtually no carbohydrates, suggested a person start his or her diet by eating only 15 to 20 grams carbohydrates a day for several weeks and slowly adding more, working up to a maintenance level of between 25 and 90. He advised that the maintenance level of carbohydrate intake is determined by the dieter's individual resistance to weight loss. The higher the resistance, the lower the carbohydrate maintenance allotment needs to be.

Other more moderate plans suggest a daily carbohydrate intake of 90 to 100 grams. Another recommends between 125 to 180 grams per day. The most liberal suggests that eating up to 250 grams is fine. In this book, we use the range of between 25 to 45 grams per meal. But the recipes will work well for your target daily carb totals.

Carb Count Consensus

We calculated the carbohydrate counts of the recipes using the website, http://caloriecount.about.com/cc/recipe_analysis. This gives us a clear and accurate tally of nutritional elements per serving of each recipe.

But even using the most advanced tools for nutritional analysis, the carbohydrate count of a recipe can't be totally precise and exact. The carbohydrate count of an orange depends on where it was grown and how long it was ripened on the vine. A medium orange is an inexact description at best. How thick is the skin? How much actual fruit is in the orange? We don't have any way of knowing these things. So the calculations are based on averages.

If you use the amounts of ingredients specified in the recipes and eat the recommended serving amounts or less, you will be eating low carb.

The Bottom Line on Carbohydrates

At the beginning of each recipe, we give you the *net carbohydrate count* of each serving, and the amount of fiber.

DEFINITION

The **net carbohydrate count** is the amount of available carbohydrates in a serving. This number is calculated by subtracting the amount of dietary fiber in grams from the carbohydrate count of the serving.

HOT POTATO

No-carb and very low-carb diets can be harmful to your health. You could be at risk for damaging your kidneys and impairing kidney function. If you have a history of low kidney function or have high blood pressure, diabetes, or are older than age 65, you are most at risk.

Not Going to Extremes

Beware of eating plans and diets that are no carb or virtually no carb. Eating that way for more than a couple weeks can jeopardize your health. You need carbohydrates for your health. They aren't bad for you; in fact, many forms of them are positively wonderful for you. Vegetables and fruits are healthful, while starchy carbs in large quantities can be harmful.

As a nation and now as a world, we are overeating starchy and sugary carbohydrates and under-eating healthy vegetables and fruits. Every fast-food restaurant, virtually every processed packaged food at the store, and every pizza joint loads us up with carbohydrates. Bread sticks, bagels, hamburger buns, french fries, and thick crusts go down so easily and wreak havoc with our weight and blood sugar levels, and our insulin levels.

Be sure to eat enough carbohydrates to maintain your health but not so much that you gain weight, increase inflammation, and worsen any health concerns. Your body needs the carbohydrates in vegetables and fruits. Our government recommends that we eat a minimum of 5 and preferably 10 servings of fruits or vegetables a day.

You can meet these recommendations eating low carb, but it is virtually impossible to do this eating no carb. Check out the vegetable, side salads, and fruit chapters. We placed special emphasis on making sure you can prepare fabulous vegetable and fruit side dishes that give your body the vitamins, phytonutrients, and antioxidants it needs, always taking into consideration the *glycemic index* of each recommended food.

DEFINITION

The **glycemic index** is the measurement of how fast a specific carbohydrate causes a rise in a person's blood sugar level. The higher the number on the glycemic index, the faster the rise in blood sugar. The Appendix contains glycemic index values for the carbohydrates used in our recipes. For a complete listing of the glycemic index of specific carbohydrates, go to www.glycemicindex.com. For a list of the net carbs, fiber, and protein for the recipes in this book, check out idiotsguide.com/lowcarbmeals.

> **TABLE TALK**
>
> When a person eats a high-glycemic food, blood sugar spikes. As a result, the pancreas gland, in a sense, overreacts and secretes more insulin than the body needs to lower the blood sugar. Leftover insulin causes the body to store yet more fat and makes the person hungry again soon afterward. This can lead to insulin resistance, inflammation, and serious health concerns such as diabetes, autoimmune disorders, and cancer.

Not All Carbs Are Created Equal

Years and years ago, when people, mostly dieters, started counting carbohydrates, it was easy. Plenty of carbohydrate counter books listed the counts. Dieters would plan their eating day simply by adding up carbs. If they wanted to eat a donut, they could, without guilt, simply by rearranging their feeding plan for the day.

Things aren't so easy today because we know more, much more. We know that fruits and vegetables are friends. We know we need to eat 5 to 10 servings of fruits and vegetables a day for health and well-being, not to mention dietary fiber.

We also know that not all carbohydrates are created equal. A donut is quite different from broccoli in how a person's blood sugar levels rise. So counting carbohydrates gets a bit challenging, if you will. Here's what you need to know:

- A carb is still a carb, and you count carb grams the same as before.

- The quality of the food containing the carbohydrates makes a difference. Eating low-glycemic carbohydrates is best for health and weight loss.

The glycemic index is a compilation of how different carbs affect a person's body. Actual scientific studies were conducted on hundreds of people. They were given different carbs to eat, and afterward, their blood sugar levels were tested.

The studies showed that some carbs made blood sugar levels spike. They are called high glycemic. And some didn't; those are called low glycemic. Some carbs are moderate glycemic because they raised blood sugar levels somewhat but didn't spike them. The carbohydrates that didn't spike blood sugar levels, the low-glycemic ones, are the best carbs to eat.

Low-glycemic carbohydrates are beneficial for those interested in eating low carb for weight loss, diabetes, high blood pressure, heart disease, inflammation, and so on.

Glycemic Index in Short

The glycemic index only measures foods that are carbohydrates, so you won't find meat or fats in the glycemic index list. The following categories are based on the general ranking of carbohydrates according to the glycemic index. For the sake of simplicity, we have categorized carbohydrates into four broad categories to help explain the glycemic index.

- Highest in the glycemic index ranking are starches that include wheat, rice, corn, white potatoes, and products made from them such as bagels, cereal, and pastas. These products range from about 70 up to 165 and are considered high glycemic. Sweet potatoes and yams aren't included here, as their glycemic index count is low.

- Sugars are rated lower, with sucrose, or table sugar, at 68. Sugars are considered moderate glycemic. This category includes natural sugars such as honey and molasses. These range from about 56 to 69. Eat these moderately, if at all.

- Fruits are low- to moderate-glycemic foods. This group includes apples, berries, oranges, peaches, pears, and other fruits, and rates range from about 30 to 50. Fifty-five or less is considered low glycemic.

- Vegetables are generally low glycemic and range from about 10 to 40. Broccoli, green beans, yams, sweet potatoes, cauliflower, and most other vegetables are in this group. As these contain the most vitamins and antioxidants, eat these often.

The carbohydrates with the lowest glycemic index values are best to eat. They help keep your blood sugar on an even keel. So broccoli is better than a donut, table sugar is somewhat better than a bagel, an apple is better than sugar, etc., even if the carb counts are exactly the same. Often the lower-glycemic foods have more nutritional value.

For day-to-day eating, choose from fruits and vegetables. Save the starches for eating occasionally, if at all. You can find a short list of the glycemic index of carbohydrate ingredients in this book in the Appendix.

Cooking Low Glycemic

The glycemic index is brilliant in that it's comprised of experiments done on actual people. It's not merely "test-tube" research. It shows how different carbohydrates actually affect real people. No prior studies have quantified results like the glycemic index. The studies have required lots of effort over years with willing volunteers.

The glycemic index works for isolated foods such as rice, but it doesn't work for combinations of foods. The very fact that the foods are combined changes the way the body reacts to them. For instance, we know that if you combine rice with a fat, such as butter, the glycemic count of the rice is lower than before. We know that if you make a brownie recipe with 5 eggs and plenty of butter, the affect of the sugar in the brownie isn't the same as if a person ate the same amount of sugar all by itself. The eggs and butter lower the glycemic effect of the sugar. If a meal contains an acidic-tasting food, like a vinaigrette salad dressing, the glycemic index effect of the whole meal is lower.

What we don't know is by how much. The only way to know the glycemic count of a recipe, that is, of a combination of ingredients, is to run the same scientific tests. No one, as of today, knows how to compute the glycemic index of a recipe with a combination of ingredients. That would require elaborate research tests on willing volunteers and could take years.

This is our solution for using the glycemic index. We chose to use ingredients that are mostly low to moderate glycemic, with a bias toward low glycemic. For example, we offer you multiple recipes for baked yams but only one for white potatoes. In the bread recipes, we use very little wheat but include other low-glycemic flours and proteins.

The ingredients in the recipes, for the most part, are already low glycemic. So you can make these recipes knowing that your eating is comfortably low to moderate glycemic.

The Least You Need to Know

- Eating healthy comfort-type foods makes for successful low-carb eating.
- Blending carbohydrate counts with glycemic index information best supports your wellness and weight-loss efforts.
- Calculating carbohydrate counts is inexact but close.
- The net carbohydrate count gives you the true bottom line on carbs.
- Eating the serving size amount listed with each recipe helps you calculate your carb intake accurately.

Meal Planning the Low-Carb Way

In This Chapter

- Eating a well-balanced diet
- Meeting your daily carbohydrate requirements
- Adding in comfort foods
- Planning your daily eating
- Understanding portions

There was a time when eating low carb meant consuming massive amounts of meat—steaks swimming in butter, chicken with the skin on, pounds of bacon—and practically nothing else. Those of us who tried the all-protein-and-fat way would awaken in the middle of the night to raid, not the refrigerator, but the breadbox. We craved bread so much it hurt. Not only that, we were bored silly eating such a one-dimensional diet.

Yes, we love steak, but too much of a good thing became a nightmare ... which could only be soothed and comforted by a sneaky midnight bread raid. Although, come to think of it, mashed potatoes or cookies also worked well to fill the void created by our meat-focused eating regimen.

Neither man nor woman was meant to live on meat alone. The focus of this chapter is to show you how to achieve that necessary balance. When we don't get balance in our day-to-day eating, our bodies and spirits pay the price. That's not the way low-carb eating should be. It's time to return to a balanced diet by eating proteins, fats, and enough carbohydrates to control your carbohydrate cravings. You'll more likely attain ideal health, vitality, and size.

Brief History of Low-Carb Eating

Low-carb eating might appear to be a modern phenomenon started a couple decades ago by a few popular diet books. However, its origins are much earlier than that—in fact, millions of years earlier. We are talking about our prehistoric ancestor, the "caveman." Whether these people lived in caves, jungles, or on open savannas, our ancient ancestors just naturally ate low carb.

Hunter-gatherers didn't raise crops or possess domesticated animals. Their diet consisted of meats, fish, eggs, vegetables, fruits, nuts, seeds, and honey. Quite simply, there wasn't anything else to eat. And there certainly weren't any grocery stores offering prepackaged Oreos!

In fact, prehistoric hunter-gatherers didn't have milk or cheese, either. There were no domesticated animals to milk, and, undoubtedly, just the thought of milking an untamed woolly mammoth mama was terrifying. Yes, the caveman and woman ate fruits and honey that had some carbohydrates. But prehistoric man never ate enough high-glycemic carbohydrates to contract the diabetes or insulin resistance that is so common today.

Only in the recent history of mankind, within the past 5,000 to 10,000 years, has man eaten cereal grains. Today foods made from refined cereal grains and sugar are available on virtually every city and suburban street corner around the world. People conveniently eat these high-carb foods in place of other more nutritious and health-giving foods in both affluent and developing countries.

In eating low carb, you are actually going back to your primitive roots and eating the foods that have sustained mankind for millions of years.

Well-Balanced Eating

The most important thing to know is that you can eat a balanced diet and eat low carb. They are completely consistent. You already know that a well-balanced diet can't include mounds of mashed potatoes, thick-crust pizza, a submarine sandwich, and a big plate of pasta all in the same day. That's called carbohydrate loading. Perhaps you've eaten this way in the past, and by now you know there's got to be a better way.

Eating in balance means eating the best ratio of fats to proteins to carbs. Ideally, every meal and every snack should contain:

- Less than 30 percent fats. Fats include butter, oils, and the fats in meat, sea-food, fish, eggs, and cheese.

- About 30 to 40 percent proteins. Complete proteins come from the animal world and include meat, fish, cheese, eggs, and seafood. Incomplete proteins come from vegetables, notably in soy, other legumes, and grains.

- About 30 to 40 percent carbohydrates. Fruits, vegetables, sugars, milk, and starches have the fewest carbs and still meet your daily carb allotment, so choose those.

Eating in balance is easy when you understand how to plan meals and know which foods to keep around for snacks and meal preparation.

Nutritional Factors: The "Best"

Some proteins, fats, and carbohydrates are better for you nutritionally than others. So let's review the best choices you can make for each category.

Fats

In this cookbook, we have used healthy and natural fats as ingredients in the recipes, such as butter and cold expeller-pressed oils. The oils include mostly olive oil and walnut oil. The only exception is a recipe for a spinach salad that uses bacon fat in the dressing.

We haven't used man-made fats that could contain carbohydrates as fillers.

One important group of fats isn't listed as an ingredient in any of the recipes. We're talking about the *essential fatty acids (EFAs)*. Your body needs EFAs for health. You get essential fatty acids when you eat cold-water fish like salmon. You can also supplement your intake with EFAs purchased from a health food store.

DEFINITION

Essential fatty acids, also called omega-3's, are fats that the body needs for health and well-being. Your body can't manufacture these nutrients from the foods it eats, and, thus, it must get them directly from foods, such as cold-water fish or from supplements like cod liver oil. These fats are designated "essential" by the government.

Protein

The best sources of *complete protein* are animal products such as meat, fish, seafood, cheese, and eggs. Animal products contain all nine essential amino acids that the body needs for health and life every day, which makes them complete proteins. All the main course dishes in this cookbook are made with complete proteins.

> **DEFINITION**
>
> **Complete proteins** contain a full complement of the nine essential amino acids the body must get through food. The only single sources of complete protein are animal products, such as fish, seafood, meat, eggs, and cheese.

To calculate how much protein you need every day, divide your weight in pounds by 2. You need that many grams complete protein. If you weigh 150 pounds, then you need 75 grams complete protein a day. This calculation is a rule of thumb, and you may find that you need somewhat less or more based on your activity levels.

For a low-carb eating plan, vegetable proteins, such as legumes and grains, may not be able to meet your amino-acid needs. Vegetable proteins are "incomplete proteins," lacking one or more of the nine essential amino acids. Each needs to be combined with another incomplete protein to give your body the full daily complement of amino acids.

The foods most often used in "food-combining" are legumes and grains. Because both are high in carbohydrates, food combining doesn't work well for low-carb eating. Eating enough beans and grains to get your daily allotment of protein significantly overloads you with carbohydrates.

Carbohydrates

To determine which types of carbohydrates to eat, you need to consider your body's nutritional needs. First and foremost, your body needs anywhere from 5 to 10 servings of fruits and vegetables a day. Does that sound like way too much food? It isn't if you put it into perspective. Half of a large-size apple or one small apple is one serving. So if you eat a large apple for breakfast, that counts as two servings. As a rule of thumb, one serving is $\frac{1}{2}$ cup cooked vegetable or one cup raw.

Here's the healthiest way to use your carb allotment:

- First, eat at least 5 servings vegetables and fruits. If your carb count allows, eat up to 10 servings.

- Next, if you have any carbohydrates left in your daily allotment after you've eaten the fruits and vegetables, choose a favorite food you especially enjoy and eat some of it. You'll find some in the bread, grains, dessert, and chocolate chapters of this book.

The Need for Starches

Nutritionally speaking, your body doesn't need starches or sugars outside the natural sugar in fruit. This means that your body doesn't require such foods as white potatoes, wheat, rice, corn, or table sugar. It doesn't even need chocolate!

Your body can get all the carbohydrate nutrition it requires from eating fruits and vegetables. Vitamins, minerals, and antioxidants are abundant in fruits and vegetables, and many are even exclusive to fruits and vegetables. That means you can't get them from starches and sugars.

Although your body doesn't need starches and sugars, they add interest, texture, and variety to our meals. If you had to give up starches and refined sugars totally, you could live just fine and be very healthy. Fortunately, you don't need to. And you don't have to as long as you make them a minor part of your eating plan.

TABLE TALK

In this cookbook, you'll find many recipes and all the chapters in Part 6 devoted to comfort foods. Chapter 22 gives you bread recipes, Chapter 23 covers grains, Chapter 24 has desserts, and Chapter 25 presents chocolate. Yes, you can have wonderful treats and happily eat low carb.

Putting Together Meals

So how do you actually put together a low-carb meal? Fortunately, you'll find it quite straightforward. Here's what to do:

- Choose a main course from Chapters 4 through 16.

- If the recipe contains vegetables and fruits, you'll count them as 1 or 2 of your 5 to 10 servings for the day.

- If the recipe doesn't include vegetables or fruits, include two servings of fruits and vegetables with that meal.

It's really just that simple. With this plan in its most basic form, you'll consume ample complete protein, and you'll eat about two servings of vegetables and fruits each meal for a total of six for the day. You really don't need to be concerned about getting enough dietary fat. You can assume that adequate fat will be included in the main dishes and any additional butter or oil used in the recipes.

Don't Eat This Way

Recently a famous actress was in the news discussing her struggle to gain 30 pounds in 6 weeks for her next movie. Her eating program was so loaded with high-carb foods that would make even a carb junkie shudder at what she consumed! Take a look at her eating plan:

- **Breakfast:** A Big Mac with large fries, scones with gravy, and a high-fat milkshake

- **Lunch:** Pizza, peanut butter with chips, and donuts

- **Dinner:** Spaghetti with meat sauce with a side of mashed potatoes and butter

Eating like this would make anyone gain 30 pounds quickly. Imagine how many carbs she was eating each meal, let alone each day! Her eating plan had no fruits and vegetables. Why? Because they would have stalled or thwarted her weight gain!

What a great example! Just eat exactly the opposite of how this actress ate to reach your personal size and health goals. You'll be eating in balance and eating low carb.

Meal Recommendations

Let's take a closer look at what does and doesn't work for low-carb meals and also for snacks.

Breakfast

Works:

- Bacon, eggs, and fruit.

- Egg and cheese omelet with vegetables.

- Ham, salmon, chicken, steak, or pork chops with vegetables and fruits.

- Fast-food egg and sausage "burger" without the bread, plus orange juice.

Doesn't work:

- Cereal and milk. Not enough protein, no fruits and veggies, and too much starch.

- Yogurt with granola and fruit. Not enough protein and too many carbohydrates.

- Bagel with cream cheese. Not enough protein, too much starch, no veggies or fruits.

- Danish and coffee. Need we say more?

Lunch

Works:

- Main dish salad. Plenty of veggies, protein. Even the ones from a fast-food restaurant are good.

- Cheese and egg main dish with salad or fruit.

- Meat or fish sandwich on one slice of bread from bread recipe in Chapter 22.

- Meat, cheese, and vegetable rollups.

- Tuna fish salad eaten with a fork and fruit or with crackers from Chapter 22.

Doesn't work:

- Submarine sandwich with potato chips.

- Corn dog. But add some fruit, and this is marginally passable.

- Fettuccine Alfredo with salad. Enough vegetables, but not enough protein and way too many carbs.

- Burger, fries, and a soft drink.

Dinner

Works:

- Roast beef or steak with asparagus and hollandaise sauce, plus salad.

- Meatloaf with Mock Mashed Potatoes and salad.

- Fried chicken minus the skin with coleslaw and fruit.

- Clam mushroom chowder and a tossed romaine salad with capers and salami.

Doesn't work:

- Pizza. To make this work, eat the topping and discard the crust, then add a big salad.

- Pasta primavera with salad. Has virtually no complete protein and possibly few vegetables. Pasta will likely add too many carbs to your daily intake.

- Salsa, chips, and guacamole. Has the veggies, but where's the protein? Too many chips equal too many carbs.

- Spaghetti with meat sauce and salad. Chances are good the carb count is too high unless you serve spaghetti squash in place of the pasta.

Snacks

These don't need to have the same portions of proteins, carbs, and fats as a meal, but they need to be low carb.

Works (all the snack recipes in this book):

- Chicken liver pâté.

- Parmesan crackers.

- Pork on a stick.

- A serving of trail mix.

- Rosemary nuts.

- Fruit with nut butter.

- Low-carb cookies from Chapter 24.

Doesn't work:

- Regular cookies from the store.

- Diet-soda soft drink and popcorn.

- Chips and salsa.

- Cheese and crackers. Instead of regular crackers, use slices of vegetables or simply hold the crackers and eat the cheese. Or use the cracker recipe in Chapter 22.

As you can tell from reading through these lists, what works is eating a balanced diet that is light on the starches. Successful low-carb eating requires you to adopt a different way of thinking about food.

Thinking of Eating

It can be quite a shock when a person first starts eating low carb. It's a shock to your eating habits, a shock to your mind, and certainly a shock to your nervous system. Every part of your body and being wants to know where the donuts are. You may be wondering how you can outsmart low-carb eating.

Until you actually experience the good feelings that come from eating low carb and until the donut cravings have subsided, you may be uncomfortable. But once the good feelings kick in, eating low carb will seem like a natural way to live.

When first starting to eat low carb, make it easy on yourself. Don't spend too much time anticipating food and eating. In that way eating becomes less emotional. Not that you won't enjoy the eating and the preparation, but you won't have time to get caught up in feeling deprived or unsatisfied.

Being deprived of your normal starchy comfort foods can make you feel as if someone just stole your favorite teddy bear. Therein lies the problem. If eating were simply a way to sustain life and provide good health, what you eat wouldn't matter much. You'd just eat at meals and then get on with doing more interesting and rewarding activities. But eating is so much more than just chewing and swallowing. Eating is the fulfillment of a sensory and emotional expectation.

The Scorecard

At the beginning of every recipe, we have included a scorecard to let you know the carbohydrate and protein count of a serving. Here's what you might find on the scorecard:

- Net carbohydrates. This number represents the amount of usable carbohydrates in a serving. This is total carbs minus dietary fiber.

- Total fiber in grams.

- Total protein in grams.

All the nutritional counts for the recipes are as accurate as possible. The actual carbohydrate and protein counts of the food you prepare can vary based on the size, ripeness, and type of ingredients you use. Be sure to eat the recommended serving size, and overall, your carb and protein counts will be very close to those listed with the recipe.

TABLE TALK

The scorecard for a recipe may not contain all the information listed here. For example, some recipes don't contain fiber or protein, so we have omitted those items.

Understanding Portions

Serving sizes in restaurants have become larger every year. Super-size fast-food meals are now the norm and no longer used to gain a marketing advantage. People are accustomed to eating lots of food—in fact, lots and lots of food—way more than the human body requires.

One wonderful, though sometimes hidden aspect of low-carb eating is that it tends to replace super-size meals with right-size meals. Grain-based foods—just think of bread, cake, and spaghetti—are precisely the kinds of foods we tend to overeat. Most of us who switch to low-carb eating just naturally tend to eat less.

The net carb count of each recipe in the scorecard is directly related to the recommended serving size. Your successful low-carb eating depends on eating the recommended amount or less.

The Least You Need to Know

- A balanced diet includes appropriate amounts of carbohydrates, protein, and fats.
- Consume vegetables and fruits in your daily carbohydrates before eating starches, treats, and snacks.
- Find ways to put together healthy nutritionally balanced meals.
- Use the nutritional counts at the beginning of each recipe to tally your intake of net carbohydrates, fiber, and protein.

Cooking the Low-Carb Way

In This Chapter

- Thinking as a low-carb cook
- Stocking a low-carb pantry
- Intelligently selecting ingredients

Cooking low-carb meals isn't much different than cooking as you've always cooked. You'll use the same techniques as before. Most likely, you'll be cooking with more fruits and vegetables, perhaps more meat, and fewer starchy ingredients, but other than that, preparation methods are the same and the cooking and baking methods are similar.

You already know how to cook, so you can easily cook low carb. The main differences won't be in your preparation methods; they are in how you think about ingredients and the combination of ingredients, which is the subject of this chapter. You won't whip up desserts using regular wheat flour, sugar, and eggs, but you still whip up desserts. You still fix a delicious Italian meat sauce, but instead of serving it over boiled spaghetti or linguine, you serve it over spaghetti squash.

You will still delight in preparing and serving good food that you, your family, and your friends still ooh and aah over.

Preparing a Low-Carb Kitchen

Your pantry may be due for a low-carb makeover. You don't need to toss out everything in the pantry and start all over again. But you'll use certain ingredients such as sugar and flour less frequently and in smaller quantities than before.

You'll keep more perishable foods in the vegetable crisper and use more eggs, butter, and olive oil. Do some kitchen shelf clearing as a way to make space for your new way of eating. We assume that low-carb eating is not a fad for you, but rather a whole new way of eating, cooking, and living.

You can toss some foods in your pantry. Here's what you can get rid of:

- Any vegetable oils that aren't *cold expeller-pressed*.
- Processed and preprepared convenience foods that have more than 25 grams carbohydrates per serving.
- Check the nutritional label on packaged low-fat products, such as salad dressings and mayonnaise. If they have lots of carbs, toss them out.
- High-carb snacks such as breads, crackers, cheese bites, and popcorn.
- Sugar-filled sodas.

DEFINITION

Cold expeller-pressed oil retains the healthy character of vegetable oils, such as olive oil and canola oil. Often oils are pressed using heat which destroys many nutrients and can compromise the taste of the oils. Check the labels to make sure you're purchasing the healthiest oils.

If in doubt, keep the food item. If you're really attached to your favorite junk food, don't toss it. Keep it around and eat it sparingly, being sure to add in the carbs to your daily count.

TABLE TALK

Keeping a daily carb journal will motivate you to avoid mindless snacking and late-night kitchen raids, plus help in pre-planning your daily menus per your daily carb allotment.

Low-Carb Ingredients

Using regular grocery-store ingredients makes low-carb cooking much easier and actually less expensive. You don't need to spend hours driving from store to store searching for just the right ingredients—virtually all the ingredients in these recipes can be purchased at a large chain grocery store. You may need to make a trip to the local health food store for some of the ingredients but not many.

Sugars

Although there are plenty of artificial sugars available, we've found that plain table sugar, sucrose, works just fine for low-carb cooking. It tastes good and leaves no aftertaste. It works perfectly in baked goods, meaning it browns beautifully and doesn't deteriorate with heat.

The American Diabetes Association (ADA) approves of regular table sugar as a sweetener for diabetics. The ADA suggests counting total carbohydrate intake rather than avoiding sugar. Small amounts of sugar are acceptable, provided that the daily carb intake is within a safe range. They recommend that a person on a 1,600-calorie-per-day food plan can eat about 200 grams carbohydrates per day.

We chose not to use artificial sweeteners in our recipes because safety and health controversies surround virtually all artificial sugars. We decided to avoid the controversy by using what we know works—regular table sugar.

If you're comfortable using a sugar substitute (such as sucralose or Truvia), you can use it in the recipes. The sugars listed here are all moderate glycemic, meaning that they only moderately stimulate a rise in blood sugar. When consumed in serving-size amounts found in the recipes, they're satisfying and great to use for low-carb cooking.

- **Table sugar.** We use as little as needed to give you good taste. Our recipes with sugar generally have fewer than 20 grams carbohydrates per serving.

- **Molasses.** Choose either light or dark, based on your personal preference. Molasses gives a wonderful "brown sugar" taste with fewer carbs than brown sugar.

- **Brown sugar.** Be sure to measure it unpacked.

- **Honey.** This all-natural sweetener is sweeter than table sugar and excellent for adding sweetness with fewer carbs.

Wheat, Pastas, and Grains

Here's an easy formula to remember: refined grains = lots of carbs. Yep. It may not be what you want to know, but you're better off confronting this simple fact directly.

Grains and grain flours are naturally high in carbs. And unfortunately, there's no magical way—at least none we know of—to make them naturally have fewer carbs.

But don't despair. They can be used in recipes in small amounts so you get their taste and texture without all the carbs. Some of our recipes use grain-based ingredients in small amounts, although most don't. Here are some key points:

- Many of our dessert recipes forego refined wheat flours entirely. Instead we use nut flours. They are out-of-this-world delicious. Our unsuspecting friends love the taste and never have a clue we left out the wheat flour. Nut flours have very few carbs, if any.

- In place of high-carb spaghetti or fettuccine, we use spaghetti squash or grated vegetables, such as zucchini. The taste is quite wonderful, and using vegetables in place of grain pastas adds more servings of nutrient-packed vegetables to your daily food intake.

- In place of lasagna noodles, we use long slices of zucchini. The zucchini gives you another vegetable serving, it's low carb, and it easily absorbs the flavors of the lasagna sauce and spices—so much so that you won't easily detect the zucchini taste.

- Some recipes produce better results with flour. For these, we use either whole-wheat flour, rice flour, or white flour in minimum quantities.

- The bread recipes use little to no wheat flour, but instead call for wheat gluten, which gives bread its stick-together-ness. Other bread ingredients include psyllium husks, oat bran, soy powder, whey powder, and, of course, the wonderful nut flours.

- For grains we use quinoa, barley, brown rice, and basmati brown rice because they are lower glycemic than other options. They still have carbs, so be sure to eat the recommended serving amount or less.

- Cornstarch is excellent for thickening sauces, and we use it in some recipes.

TABLE TALK

Make nut flours by processing whole or chopped nuts in a food processor. Purchase bulk nuts in the grocery store or health food store bins. Generally speaking, ¾ cup nuts makes 1 cup nut flour.

Potatoes

Potatoes are also a naturally high-carb food. In general, if you're going to eat low carb, you'll need to limit your potato intake and avoid recipes with potatoes. Rather than go completely without potatoes, however, we have devised recipes that let you have some. Consider these few details:

- You'll find recipes for sweet potatoes and yams, which are lower glycemic than white potatoes and have a sweeter taste.

- Cauliflower is an excellent vegetable substitute for mashed potatoes and potato salad. When prepared properly, it cooks up to have similar color and texture. When you prepare cauliflower with a little garlic, butter, or gravy, you'll find the taste and texture a viable substitute for potatoes.

- Potato skins without the insides give you the taste without the carbs.

- You can make clam chowder with mushrooms instead of potatoes. You'll never miss the potatoes when you taste this soup.

Fats

Thank goodness, you can enjoy the mouth-satisfying taste of fat when eating low carb.

- **Olive oil that is cold expeller-pressed.** In general, the darker the color of the oil, the higher it is in antioxidants.

- **Butter.** Butter heats beautifully, and nothing tastes quite like real butter. Use for sautéing, baking, and melting over steamed vegetables.

- **Walnut oils and other cold expeller-pressed oils.** You may need to shop at the health food store to find these. They are worth the price. Don't heat them, though.

- **Heated bacon fat.** You can heat it safely to use in small amounts, as in a salad dressing.

Dairy

We're not fans of low-fat or skim milk. Our recipes here call for dairy products in their full-fat versions. Why? Because low-fat dairy products usually have more carbs and when used for cooking, they don't deliver as satisfying a product. Taste matters! It's amazing how often individuals will eat a much larger quantity of a low-fat food than the regular variety and, in the process, consume more calories and sometimes more fat.

- **Heavy cream.** Find the thickest, richest cream you can. Go beyond regular whipping cream if heavy cream is available.

- **Milk.** Use whole milk.

- **Cheeses.** Regular grocery store–quality cheeses work well in these recipes. Save yourself time and use the pregrated cheeses that come in resealable bags when you can.

- **Eggs.** Use large eggs.

If your dietary needs limit fat, then by all means, use the low-fat version in the recipes. You'll be enjoying great taste, lower amounts of fat, and the benefits of eating low carb.

Fruits and Vegetables

Make friends with the produce aisle! Vegetables and fruits get heavy emphasis in our cookbook because of their value to your low-carb eating plan. Even though fruit may get a bad rap for containing carbs, they are much lower in carbs than junk food, fast food, and sugared sodas, not to mention french fries! Plus fruits are loaded with valuable vitamins, minerals, phytochemicals, and antioxidants.

There simply aren't any substitutes for fruits and vegetables; fortunately, you don't need substitutes. Purchase produce fresh or frozen and eat about two servings each meal. Yes, that's two servings for breakfast, lunch, and dinner. You really can't go wrong eating them, but you can definitely go wrong if you don't eat them.

The Least You Need to Know

- You can make your pantry low carb by switching out some items for their low-carb counterparts.
- Most ingredients for low-carb cooking are available locally.
- Regular cooking ingredients can produce great low-carb meals.
- Grain-based ingredients and potatoes tend to be high carb, but most other ingredients are not.
- Eating smaller portions of low-carb foods will leave you satisfied without overeating.

Breakfasts and Lunches

The first meal of the day, breakfast, can supply you with plenty of energy for the rest of your day. Yes, eating a good low-carb breakfast boosts your metabolism and sets the stage for having a good high-energy day.

Preparing a quick low-carb breakfast is a high priority in our time-challenged lives. You no longer need to skip breakfast. These recipes give you countless ways to grab or prepare a great breakfast—fast and easy. The Leisurely Breakfasts chapter has many recipes for enjoying a late-morning or weekend brunch.

Pack a delicious low-carb lunch for work or outings and avoid the standard high-carb sandwich and chips. Instead, savor meat and cheese rollups, trail mix, and homemade nut butters with fruit.

Breakfast on the Run

In This Chapter

- Eating our most important meal
- Getting enough complete protein
- Rushing to get out the door

Ah, donuts! We've loved them all, but we also all know they aren't exactly what the nutritionist—or our mother!—would recommend as the ideal way to begin a day. Plus, they are very high in carbohydrates.

You've heard that a "good breakfast" is your most important meal of the day. Whether or not you eat a good breakfast can determine your overall energy levels and even your moods for the day. A good breakfast is a key way to avoid sudden drops in energy and cravings for a sugar lift come mid-morning. So what constitutes a "good breakfast"? The answer is simple—a low-carb one.

A low-carb breakfast gives you the protein, fat, and enough carbs to stoke your metabolism and get your fat-burning system running on high speed.

But figuring out what to eat for breakfast takes forethought and some planning, especially on those days when you're rushing to get yourself and your family out the door in the mornings. That's why this chapter is devoted to solving the very real problem of how to eat this most important of meals when you're in a rush.

Rise and Shine

Skipping breakfast isn't a great idea. In fact, it's a terrible idea. Your body needs food to "break fast," that is, to restore itself following the long fasting period since supper the night before. Most likely a person hasn't eaten any food for 8 to 12 hours by the time he rises and shines. You want not only to rise but also to shine, and breakfast helps you do just that.

In breaking your fast, you jump-start the body's energy-making machine for the whole day:

- Your metabolism goes into high gear when you eat a good, balanced breakfast.

- Because your metabolism cues fat-burning, a good, balanced breakfast helps you stay at your ideal size and even lose weight.

- Eating a good, balanced breakfast helps keep your energy levels high all day long and into the evening.

- As an extra bonus, eating a good, balanced breakfast can keep your moods lifted, your disposition friendly, and your mind and body productive.

"All this from breakfast?" you ask. Absolutely!

A Good, Balanced Breakfast

A good, balanced breakfast provides you with a balanced meal of protein, fat, and carbohydrates. We're not talking about a lot of carbohydrates, but some, because, as you know, you need some carbs for health and energy.

So let's look specifically at what's in a good, low-carb breakfast:

- High-quality complete protein that comes from meat, fish, eggs, or cheese. On the average, you need 15 to 20 grams of animal protein at each meal, breakfast included. Men may need more.

- At least one serving of either fruits or vegetables, preferably two servings.

- A modest amount of fat. Yes, fat is absolutely necessary for a healthy diet and a healthy you. You'll get some fat in the eggs, meat, and cheese, plus the butter used for cooking. Fat gives you energy to burn.

As you have probably noticed, cereal just doesn't make the grade, ditto for yogurt and granola, and certainly a Danish or bagel washed down with coffee doesn't qualify. So what does?

Think of traditional old-fashioned breakfasts with ham and eggs, omelets, fresh fruit, steak and eggs, or fish. Or what about the sort of thing one might find at an English country breakfast (eggs, bacon, sausages, toast)? Now, that's a good breakfast.

TABLE TALK

The simple truth is this: what you eat for breakfast can be anything you want. Just because other folks eat a Danish with a cup of coffee doesn't mean you need to. Gosh, you can cook up green beans or asparagus for breakfast if you want. You can fry up a steak or some halibut. How about having a little leftover barbecue? If you enjoy it, that's what counts.

Food That's Ready Fast, Not Fast Food

A leisurely breakfast can be hard to manage in a busy household. Too often there's not enough time, and getting breakfast prepared and eaten when you're rushed is challenging. But it can be lots easier when you know how.

So even though your mornings are rushed, there's still time for a great breakfast. Just get creative. And never forget how important a good breakfast is for your health—and for your family's. Rise and shine with these quick breakfasts.

Microwave Bacon

Yield:	Serving size:	Prep time:	Cook time:
4 servings	2 slices	5 minutes	8 minutes
Each serving has:			
0 g carbohydrate	0 g fiber	5 g protein	

8 slices bacon

1. Place a layer of white paper towels on a microwaveable baking dish. Arrange bacon slices on the paper towels so that each slice is flat, but they can be touching. Cover with another layer of paper towels.

2. Place in a microwave on high for 8 minutes or until bacon is done.

3. To cook more bacon, you can add another layer of bacon on top of the paper towels. Then cover with one more layer of paper towels. Add 1 minute cooking time for each additional slice of bacon.

Variation: Cooked salami, as a substitute for bacon, is great with eggs for breakfast or crumbled into a tossed salad. To cook salami, arrange it in a baking dish as you did the bacon. Depending on the thickness of the salami, cook 30 seconds to 1 minute per slice.

RECIPE FOR SUCCESS

This method makes great bacon and doesn't smell up the house as much as frying bacon does. You also don't have to dispose of the grease in the pan—simply toss the paper towels in the trash. Use paper towels that are made without dyes, inks, and perfumes and are considered hypo-allergenic.

Granola

Yield:	Serving size:	Prep time:	Cook time:
18 servings	½ cup	10 minutes	1 hour
Each serving has:			
15 g carbohydrate	4 g fiber	10 g protein	

½ cup butter (1 stick)

2½ cups old-fashioned rolled oats

1 cup sunflower seeds

¾ cup wheat germ

1 cup flaked coconut, unsweetened

½ cup walnuts, chopped

1 cup pumpkin seeds

½ cup wheat bran

¼ cup golden raisins

¼ cup dried cranberries

½ cup whole almonds

¼ cup honey

1. Preheat the oven to 250°F.

2. Melt butter in a large, shallow roasting pan on top of the stove. Remove from heat and stir in oats, sunflower seeds, wheat germ, coconut, walnuts, pumpkin seeds, wheat bran, raisins, cranberries, and almonds. Mix well.

3. Drizzle honey over mixture, and stir until well blended.

4. Place the pan in the oven, and toast for 1 hour, stirring every 15 minutes. Store in an airtight container for up to 4 months.

RECIPE FOR SUCCESS

Use this granola as a side dish for breakfast. Make the main course no-carb eggs, meat, fish, or cheese. You can have the granola on the side as a finger food, or eat it topped with some heavy cream, half-and-half, or low-carb yogurt. It's also great as a trail mix snack.

Microwave Scrambled Eggs

Yield:	Serving size:	Prep time:	Cook time:
2 servings	1½ eggs	2 minutes	3 minutes
Each serving has:			
1 g carbohydrate	0 g fiber	10 g protein	

1 TB. butter

3 large eggs

1 TB. water

Salt and pepper to taste

1. Place butter in a glass measuring cup or bowl. Microwave on high for 20 seconds.

2. Mix eggs and water into melted butter until well mixed, being certain to pierce the yolks.

3. Place container in the microwave on high for 1 minute. Stir eggs. Microwave for 1 more minute or until eggs are just a slight bit runny. Let stand 1 minute before serving. Add salt and pepper to taste.

RECIPE FOR SUCCESS

If you aren't hungry for breakfast, crack some eggs into a glass or plastic container, being sure to pierce the yolks. Add a pat of butter, and cover with the lid. Take the container to work. By the time you get there, the eggs should be well mixed. Cook mixture in a microwave when you get hungry, and you have a perfect breakfast on the run.

Hard Boiled Eggs

Yield:	Serving size:	Prep time:	Cook time:
6 servings	1 egg	5 minutes	20 minutes

Each serving has:			
< 1 g carbohydrate	0 g fiber	6 g protein	

6 large eggs, raw, in shell

1. Put eggs in a large saucepan without stacking on top of one another. Add enough water to cover tops by 1 inch. Cover the pan and rapidly bring water to a boil.

2. Remove the pan from heat, and allow it to stand, covered, for 15 minutes. Remove eggs from hot water, and immediately place them into a bowl of cold water. This helps make shells easier to remove and prevents discoloration of yolks.

3. To remove shells, tap surface of egg to crack; roll egg between hands to loosen shell; and beginning at larger end of egg, peel off shell. It may help to dip egg into the bowl of cold water to ease off shell.

TABLE TALK

Eggs have all the amino acids the body needs in the correct proportion; in fact, the egg is the basic standard against which all other protein foods are measured. Who said the egg is not a healthy food?

Make-Ahead Italian Bake

Yield:	Serving size:	Prep time:	Cook time:
6 servings	1 square	10 minutes	30 minutes

Each serving has:		
7 g carbohydrate	2 g fiber	9 g protein

1 TB. butter	$\frac{1}{4}$ tsp. cayenne
$\frac{1}{2}$ cup green onions, chopped	2 large eggs, beaten
1 cup cremini mushrooms, sliced	$\frac{1}{2}$ cup cheddar cheese, shredded
1 (14-oz.) can artichoke hearts, drained and chopped	$\frac{1}{2}$ cup Swiss cheese, shredded
$\frac{1}{2}$ tsp. dried oregano	$\frac{1}{2}$ cup Italian breadcrumbs

1. Preheat the oven to 350°F.

2. Melt butter in a skillet, and sauté onions and mushrooms. In a separate medium bowl, combine artichoke hearts with oregano, cayenne, eggs, cheddar and Swiss cheeses, and breadcrumbs; add onion and mushrooms and stir well.

3. Pour into a buttered 8-inch-square pan. Bake for 30 minutes until set.

4. Cut into 6 squares. Refrigerate leftovers for the next day.

Ham Rollups

Yield:	Serving size:	Prep time:	Cook time:
3 servings	2 rollups	10 minutes	None

Each serving has:		
3 g carbohydrate	1 g fiber	23 g protein

6 slices ham	6 TB. various fruits or vegetables, matchstick size or chopped
6 slices cheese (your favorite)	

1. Top ham slice with cheese and various small pieces of fruit or vegetables of choice. Roll up ham; place in the sandwich bags if not eaten immediately.

Suggestions for vegetables: Bell pepper, radish, celery, broccoli flowerets, raw spinach, tomato, carrot, etc.

Suggestions for fruits: Pineapple bits, apple, banana, peach, berries, dried fruits, etc.

Egg Rolls

Yield:	Serving size:	Prep time:	Cook time:
6 servings	1 egg roll	10 minutes	20 minutes
Each serving has:			
8 g carbohydrate	2 g fiber	15 g protein	

$\frac{1}{2}$ tsp. butter

6 large eggs, beaten

$1\frac{1}{2}$ cups milk

$\frac{1}{4}$ cup all purpose flour

5 green onions, thinly sliced

Salt and pepper to taste

1 cup cheddar cheese, shredded

1. Preheat the oven to 350°F.

2. Line a 10×15-inch rimmed baking sheet with aluminum foil; coat foil with butter.

3. In a large bowl, whisk together eggs, milk, flour, onions, salt, and pepper. When mixture is smooth, pour evenly onto the baking pan.

4. Bake for 12 to 15 minutes until set. Sprinkle evenly with cheese and bake 2 minutes or until cheese is melted.

5. Cool for 5 minutes. Carefully lift the foil (eggs and all) and remove from the baking pan. Starting from smaller end, roll up the eggs, jellyroll style, carefully releasing them from the foil as you roll. Slice into 1-inch pieces and serve.

RECIPE FOR SUCCESS

You can add chopped cooked ham, bacon, sausage, or vegetables to this mixture before baking. If preparing more than one, you can refrigerate the baked rolls. When ready to serve, cut and reheat. The rolls are especially delicious served with salsa!

Open-Face Canadian Bacon Sandwich

Yield:	Serving size:	Prep time:	Cook time:
2 servings	1 slice Canadian bacon and 1 egg	10 minutes	5 minutes

Each serving has:			
1 g carbohydrate	0 g fiber	14 g protein	

2 Canadian bacon rounds

2 large eggs

Salt and pepper to taste

2 slices tomato, optional

1 slice favorite cheese (cut in half)

1. Slowly warm cooked Canadian bacon in a skillet over medium heat. While meat is warming, break 1 egg into each custard cup or similar small dish. Prick yolk with a fork, season with salt and pepper if desired, cover with a paper towel, and cook in a microwave approximately 45 to 60 seconds.

2. Place each Canadian bacon round on small plate, top with egg and tomato (if desired), and cover with $\frac{1}{2}$ cheese slice. Microwave approximately 15 seconds until cheese melts.

3. Eat as an open-face sandwich.

RECIPE FOR SUCCESS

You may add additional vegetables such as mushrooms, bell pepper, chopped onion, etc. If desired, place a second round of Canadian bacon on top of cheese to make a "sandwich."

Egg Pancake

Yield:	Serving size:	Prep time:	Cook time:
1 serving	1 pancake	5 minutes	10 minutes

Each serving has:			
1 g carbohydrate	0 g fiber	13 g protein	

1 TB. butter

2 large eggs, beaten

Salt and pepper to taste

1 TB. chopped onion, bell pepper, or tomato; salsa; or chopped cooked meat

1. Melt butter in a 10-inch skillet over medium-low heat, add beaten eggs, and spread in the skillet. Cook eggs without stirring until set.

2. Invert the skillet over a plate to allow egg pancake to fall onto the plate.

3. Sprinkle with salt and pepper and chopped vegetable or meat. Roll up to eat on the run.

RECIPE FOR SUCCESS

This recipe makes a delicious hot or cold snack or even breakfast on the run.

The Least You Need to Know

- A good breakfast contains complete protein, fruits or veggies, and fat.
- Eating a good, balanced, low-carb breakfast boosts your metabolism.
- Eating a quick, healthy breakfast gives you all the nutrition you need to jump-start your day and your metabolism.
- Eat any meats, fish, eggs, and cheese you like for breakfast, but avoid traditional starch-filled breakfast foods like toast and cereal.

Chapter 5

Leisurely Breakfasts

In This Chapter

- Taking time for breakfast
- Planning the meal
- Selecting brunch ingredients

It's a cozy Saturday morning, and the paper has arrived. Now's the time to relax and enjoy cooking and eating delicious brunch fare. Of course, you can also enjoy these recipes for lunch or dinner or on any day of the week when you have the time. But there's something about a leisurely breakfast that will put a smile on everyone's face and yours, too.

In this chapter we set the stage for serving these delightful meals with soft classical music playing in the background, flowers on the table, and good china with cloth napkins.

Filled with Goodness

The ingredients in these recipes are selected specifically because they yield a low-carb entrée. Here's a list of what the recipes call for:

- **Whole-fat dairy products.** We suggest you use whole cream, cheese, and milk because substituting low-fat versions will typically increase the carbohydrate count. If you prefer, you can use low-fat dairy products.

- **Vegetables.** As best possible, choose fresh or frozen. Avoid the canned versions, as they have fewer nutrients.

- **Real butter.** Use butter substitutes if you prefer to reduce dietary cholesterol. Otherwise, go ahead and enjoy the flavor and texture of real butter.

- **Eggs.** Use large eggs. Egg substitutes are fine to use, but keep in mind they can sometimes alter your results.

- **Chicken broth.** If you don't have this on hand, you can make an acceptable substitute by using a chicken bouillon cube and water. Be sure to omit the salt in the recipe, as bouillon has plenty.

Whether cooking for family or friends, these recipes are terrific to serve to weekend guests or even before the big game. Your guests will applaud your cooking, want the recipes, and be shocked to learn that dishes that taste so good can be low carb, too.

Eggs Benedict

Yield:	Serving size:	Prep time:	Cook time:
6 servings	2 slices Canadian bacon with 1 egg	15 minutes	5 minutes
Each serving has:			
1 g carbohydrate	< 1 g fiber	27 g protein	

$\frac{1}{2}$ cup butter (1 stick)	6 large eggs
4 large egg yolks at room temperature	12 slices Canadian bacon
1 TB. fresh lemon juice	$\frac{1}{2}$ lb. spinach leaves, washed
	6 slices tomato

1. Prepare hollandaise sauce first: Melt butter in a pan or the microwave. Put egg yolks and lemon juice into a blender. Turn on the blender, and slowly pour warm butter into the blender. Whir for a couple seconds. Set aside.

2. Poach eggs using an egg poacher and follow instructions. If you don't have an egg poacher, bring an inch of water to simmer in a large skillet. Crack each egg and carefully slide the egg into the simmering water. Cover skillet for 3 minutes.

Check eggs for doneness, keeping yolks whole and partially runny. If necessary, continue to cook a minute or two longer until the eggs reach desired doneness. On each plate, place 2 slices Canadian bacon, and top with 4 to 5 spinach leaves and 1 tomato slice. Top with poached egg.

3. Spoon hollandaise sauce over eggs, and serve right away.

Variation: Substitute sliced smoked salmon for the Canadian bacon.

Ham Flan

Yield:	Serving size:	Prep time:	Cook time:
6 servings	1 wedge	20 minutes	60 minutes
Each serving has:			
2 g carbohydrate	< 1 g fiber	10 g protein	

$1\frac{1}{2}$ cups heavy cream

1 cup ham, chopped

1 TB. green onions, chopped

1 tsp. black pepper

4 large eggs

$\frac{1}{4}$ tsp. butter

1. Preheat the oven to 325°F.

2. Stirring constantly, heat cream in a saucepan over medium-low heat until small bubbles form. Remove the pan from heat, and stir in ham, green onions, and pepper.

3. Beat 1 egg in a small bowl, and slowly pour in about 2 tablespoons hot mixture; stir until combined. Beat second egg into this mixture by hand. Pour eggs into slightly cooled mixture in the saucepan. Add last 2 eggs, beating as each is added until completely combined.

4. Pour mixture into a buttered pie pan, and place in a larger pan of hot water. Bake for 45 minutes until set. Insert a clean knife into custard to be sure it is done. The knife should come out clean when thoroughly cooked. Cut into 6 wedges.

Variation: Add 1 cup of your favorite grated cheese to the hot cream and stir until it melts; then add the rest of the ingredients as instructed. This dish is just as delicious served cold and cut into wedges. It makes a great breakfast on the run or an afternoon snack.

TABLE TALK

When adding raw eggs to a hot mixture, first stir a small portion of the hot mixture into the beaten egg to warm it up. If the raw egg is dumped suddenly into the hot mixture, the protein in the egg will likely coagulate, clump, and partially cook (think scrambled).

Asparagus Tart

Yield:	Serving size:	Prep time:	Cook time:
6 servings	1 wedge	20 minutes	60 minutes
Each serving has:			
3 g carbohydrate	< 1 g fiber	11 g protein	

$1\frac{1}{2}$ cups heavy cream

1 cup Swiss cheese, grated

1 TB. red onion, diced

1 TB. bell pepper, diced

1 tsp. black pepper

1 tsp. paprika

4 large eggs

$\frac{1}{2}$ cup fresh or frozen asparagus, blanched and cut into bite-size pieces

$\frac{1}{4}$ tsp. butter

1. Preheat the oven to 325°F.

2. Stirring constantly, heat cream in a saucepan over medium-low heat until small bubbles form. Add cheese and stir continuously until melted. Remove the pan from heat, and blend in onion, bell pepper, black pepper, and paprika.

3. Beat 1 egg in a small bowl, and slowly pour in about 2 tablespoons hot mixture; stir until combined. Beat second egg into this mixture with a fork. Pour egg mixture into slightly cooled mixture in the saucepan. Add last 2 eggs, beating as each is added until completely combined.

4. Line a buttered pie pan with asparagus, and pour mixture into the pan. Place the pan into a larger pan of hot water, and bake for 45 minutes, until set.

5. Insert a clean knife into custard to be sure it is done. The knife should come out clean when thoroughly cooked. Cut into 6 wedges.

Variation: This tart is refreshing served cold and cut into wedges. It makes a great afternoon pick-me-up snack. Serve with fresh fruit or a light green salad with chopped green apples. If you are not a lover of asparagus, any vegetable may be substituted, such as $\frac{1}{2}$ cup green beans or cooked spinach. This is a great way to use leftover vegetables!

TABLE TALK

Stirring a small amount of the hot mixture into the egg helps prevent cooking the egg versus dumping the egg into the saucepan and ending up with egg drop soup!

Brunch Egg Casserole

Yield:	Serving size:	Prep time:	Cook time:
6 servings	$\frac{1}{6}$ casserole	Day before, 20 minutes	45 minutes

Each serving has:			
12 g carbohydrate	< 1 g fiber	30 g protein	

4 slices whole-wheat bread, crust removed

1 lb. ground sausage or sausage links, thinly sliced

1 cup chopped vegetable mixture, such as mushrooms, bell peppers, onions, pimento, jalapeño peppers, etc.

1 cup cheddar cheese, shredded

6 large eggs

1 tsp. dry mustard

Pepper to taste

2 cups heavy cream

1. Preheat the oven to 350°F.

2. Lightly toast bread and break into small pieces; place bread in a 9 × 13-inch buttered glass baking dish.

3. Brown sausage in a skillet over medium heat. Drain and pat with plain white paper towels. Sprinkle sausage over bread; next layer with vegetables and cheese.

4. Beat eggs with a fork in a small bowl. Add dry mustard, pepper, and cream. Beat again. Pour egg mixture evenly over all ingredients. Cover with foil and refrigerate overnight.

5. Remove the foil. Bake 45 minutes or until casserole is bubbly and lightly browned on top. Let stand 30 minutes after baking.

RECIPE FOR SUCCESS

This casserole is best when it stands 30 minutes after baking. It's a great dish to prepare ahead of time because it can be frozen in the pan before baking. Remove from the freezer and thaw overnight in the refrigerator.

Salmon Soufflé

Yield:	Serving size:	Prep time:	Cook time:
6 servings	⅙ soufflé	20 minutes	50 to 60 minutes

Each serving has:		
3 g carbohydrate	0 g fiber	19 g protein

1 (15½-oz.) can salmon, drained	½ tsp. pepper
3 TB. butter	½ tsp. dill
3 TB. flour	4 large egg whites, stiffly beaten
1 cup heavy cream	¼ tsp. butter
4 large egg yolks, beaten	

1. Preheat the oven to 350°F.

2. Drain salmon, remove skin and bones, and *flake*.

3. Melt butter in a saucepan over low heat; gradually add flour and cream, and stir until thickened.

4. Remove the pan from heat. Stir small amount of hot mixture into beaten egg yolks to keep yolks from coagulating and partially cooking. Now slowly pour egg yolks into hot mixture, stirring constantly. Cook over low heat 1 minute; add pepper, dill, and flaked salmon.

5. After egg whites are *stiffly beaten*, slowly fold salmon mixture into egg whites; lightly fold egg whites over and over until combined with salmon mixture.

6. Pour into a buttered 2-quart baking dish. Place the dish in a larger pan of hot water, and bake for 50 to 60 minutes. Serve immediately.

Variation: This soufflé makes a delightful addition to a breakfast buffet or light lunch with fresh fruit. There are almost as many variations of this soufflé as you can imagine. In place of the salmon you can add 1 cup grated cheese and stir until it melts or add 1 cup chopped spinach or chopped onions. Let your imagination run wild!

DEFINITION

To **flake** means to break up with a fork into bite-size pieces. To **stiffly beat** egg whites, use a large bowl and whip with electric mixer until peaks form and stand up straight.

Mexican Omelet

Yield:	Serving size:	Prep time:	Cook time:
2 servings	½ omelet	10 minutes	15 minutes
Each serving has:			
9 g carbohydrate	3 g fiber	15 g protein	

1 (14-oz.) can chicken broth

¼ cup onion, chopped

¼ cup bell pepper, chopped

1 clove garlic, crushed

1 (15-oz.) can tomatoes, drained and chopped

1 (4-oz.) can green chilies, chopped

4 TB. butter

4 large eggs, beaten

½ cup cheddar cheese, grated

1. To make sauce: Pour chicken broth into a skillet. Add chopped onion, bell pepper, and garlic. Simmer and add tomatoes and chilies. Cook 10 minutes.

2. While sauce simmers, heat butter in a skillet. Tilt pan so butter coats sides of pan all the way to the top to prevent omelet from sticking. Set pan over medium-low heat. Pour beaten eggs into skillet. With a spatula, push egg in from the sides to allow top, uncooked egg to run over to pan. When eggs are set on bottom, immediately add grated cheese and fold omelet in half. Cook another 5 minutes until puffed up.

3. Remove mixture from the pan, cut into 2 servings, placing ½ omelet on each plate, and pour sauce on top.

4. For additional omelets, wipe the pan with a paper towel, and repeat for next omelet. You will have enough sauce for about 3 omelets. Store unused sauce in an airtight container in the refrigerator for later use on omelets or burgers.

RECIPE FOR SUCCESS

If you prefer a spicier omelet, you can add ¼ teaspoon each cumin, chili powder, and oregano along with chopped jalapeño peppers. This makes a great luncheon dish served with fresh fruit. For fluffier, mile-high omelets, beat the egg whites separately and fold them into the yolks before pouring into the omelet pan.

German Pancakes

Yield:	Serving size:	Prep time:	Cook time:
4 servings	¼ pancake	15 minutes	3 minutes
Each serving has:			
9 g carbohydrate	0 g fiber	9 g protein	

6 large eggs	¼ cup milk
1 TB. sugar	4 TB. butter
2 TB. cornstarch	4 tsp. lemon juice
½ tsp. salt	Sprinkle confectioners' sugar
¼ cup water	

1. Beat eggs with sugar, cornstarch, salt, water, and milk. Heat 2 tablespoons butter in an omelet pan. Pour batter into the pan, and cook as a pancake.

2. Divide pancake onto 4 plates. Put $\frac{1}{2}$ tablespoon butter and 1 teaspoon lemon juice on each serving. Sprinkle lightly with confectioners' sugar.

RECIPE FOR SUCCESS

German pancakes have a slightly sweet taste, balanced with the lemony butter on top. You can also serve them with the following pancake syrup recipe and omit the lemon juice and confectioners' sugar. This will be a hit every time you serve or eat it. The pancake puffs up when cooking but usually falls before serving. The edges get lightly browned and crusty.

Pancake Syrup

Yield:	Serving size:	Prep time:	Cook time:
8 servings	2 tablespoons	5 minutes	5 minutes
Each serving has:			
10 g carbohydrate	0 g fiber	0 g protein	

1 cup water

1 cup no-sugar-added preserves (avoid those sweetened with sugar substitutes)

1. Heat water in a saucepan until bubbles appear. Slowly add preserves, stirring continuously until completely combined. Boil on medium-high heat for 5 minutes until of syrup consistency.

2. Serve warm or cold.

Easy Cheese Breakfast Soufflé

Yield:	Serving size:	Prep time:	Cook time:
6 servings	$\frac{1}{6}$ soufflé	10 minutes	35 to 40 minutes

Each serving has:		
1 g carbohydrate	0 g fiber	17 g protein

6 large eggs

1 cup heavy cream

Salt and pepper to taste

$\frac{1}{4}$ tsp. nutmeg

1 cup Swiss or cheddar cheese, grated

$\frac{1}{2}$ cup Parmesan cheese, grated

$\frac{1}{2}$ tsp. butter

1. Preheat the oven to 425°F.

2. Beat eggs until thick and light. Stir in cream, salt, pepper, and nutmeg. Fold in Swiss and Parmesan cheeses. Pour into a well-buttered $1\frac{1}{2}$-quart baking dish or a $10\frac{1}{2}$-inch ovenproof skillet.

3. Bake 35 to 40 minutes until set.

Cranberry Eggs

Yield:	Serving size:	Prep time:	Cook time:
10 servings	$\frac{1}{10}$ recipe	10 minutes	50 to 60 minutes

Each serving has:		
9 g carbohydrate	6 g fiber	5 g protein

2 large eggs

$\frac{3}{8}$ cup sugar

$\frac{1}{2}$ cup butter, melted (1 stick)

1 cup almond flour

$\frac{1}{2}$ cup pecans, chopped

1 cup whole fresh or frozen cranberries

1. Preheat the oven to 325°F.

2. Combine eggs, sugar, butter, almond flour, pecans, and cranberries. Pour into a greased baking dish. Bake 50 to 60 minutes. Serve warm.

RECIPE FOR SUCCESS

Use this as a side dish for a leisurely and special breakfast. It's great for the holidays. Add meat such as ham or bacon to balance the sweet-tart taste of this recipe and to get enough complete protein for your meal.

Crustless Quiche

Yield:	Serving size:	Prep time:	Cook time:
8 servings	$\frac{1}{8}$ casserole	15 minutes	45 minutes
Each serving has:			
3 g carbohydrate	0 g fiber	23 g protein	

$\frac{1}{2}$ cup butter (1 stick)	2 cups cottage cheese
2 TB. flour	$\frac{1}{2}$ cup ham, diced
6 large eggs	$\frac{1}{2}$ cup spinach, chopped
1 cup milk	1 tsp. baking powder
1 lb. Monterey Jack cheese, cubed	$\frac{1}{2}$ tsp. salt
1 (3-oz.) pkg. cream cheese, softened	1 tsp. sugar

1. Preheat the oven to 325°F.

2. Melt butter in a small saucepan. Add flour to saucepan and cook until smooth. Beat eggs and milk together in a small bowl, then add to the saucepan. Stir in Monterey Jack cheese, cream cheese, cottage cheese, ham, spinach, baking powder, salt, sugar, and butter-flour mixture. Stir until well blended. Pour into a well-greased 9 × 13 × 2-inch pan.

3. Bake uncovered for 45 minutes.

RECIPE FOR SUCCESS

Quiche is wonderful—and easier to make without the crust. You'll enjoy the creamy taste of the eggs and cheeses.

Eggs with Spinach

Yield:	Serving size:	Prep time:	Cook time:
6 servings	1 egg	15 minutes	30 minutes
Each serving has:			
2 g carbohydrate	< 1 g fiber	14 g protein	

2 TB. butter

2 TB. flour

2 cups heavy cream

1 tsp. white pepper

1 (10-oz.) pkg. frozen spinach, thawed and squeezed dry

6 large eggs

1 cup cheddar or mozzarella cheese, shredded

1. Preheat the oven to 350°F.

2. Heat butter in a pan and add flour, stirring constantly until thick. Add cream and pepper and stir until well blended.

3. Line bottom of a buttered oblong baking dish with spinach. Make 6 indentations in spinach, and break 1 egg into each.

4. Pour cream sauce over eggs, and sprinkle with cheese. Bake for 30 minutes.

The Least You Need to Know

- Brunch entrées are easily and naturally low carb.
- Using the specified ingredients ensures a delicious low-carb brunch.
- Add two servings of fruit and/or vegetables to each entrée for a balanced and healthy meal.
- If your brunch occasion calls for something sweet, choose from desserts and chocolate in Chapters 24 and 25.

Lunches

In This Chapter

- Choosing foods for lunch
- Thinking outside the lunch box
- Making lunches without sandwiches

A woman walked up to the counter at the local deli, and seeing that they didn't offer salads, ordered a ham and cheese sandwich, hold the bread. Without batting an eyelash, the deli owner declared, "I can do that." The paper plate she received held ham, cheese, lettuce, and a deli pickle plus mustard and mayonnaise packets.

This scene is being played out more and more—at delis, fast-food drive-thru lanes, and even at submarine sandwich shops. If a restaurant can't or won't hold the bread, some of us simply ask for a fork and knife and eat the insides of the sandwich. We put the bread on hold for ourselves. The insides of the sandwich make for a perfect lunch.

Today the more progressive, popular fast-food restaurants offer interesting and inexpensive salads filled with greens, vegetables, and chicken or beef. The trend toward low carb is now well established, and eating a low-carb lunch is easier than it's ever been. In this chapter we focus on lunch options that are quick, easy, and satisfying.

Lunch Is Important

Lunch isn't something to be taken lightly—perhaps eaten lightly, but not taken lightly. That's why we've included a chapter on lunches in this cookbook. You may need to adjust your thinking about lunch and modify a few of your well-established midday eating habits. This chapter will give you the tools you need to accomplish those goals.

Some of you who eat lunch at a restaurant every day have figured out how to eat low carb. But many folks are still stuck in the "fries and burger" rut. Or they take a lunch to work occasionally (or want to) and haven't figured out what to pack. Even eating a low-carb lunch at home can be tricky at first.

Packing low-carb lunches for the kids can be rough, too. If they want to eat at school, the prime choice is usually one basic starch or another. The entrées offered are now such things as pizza or some other fast food … hold the vegetables and fruit, which definitely is not good.

Don't despair, because a healthy lunch is important. And you don't want to skip lunch. Eating lunch keeps your energy high and can avert late-day fatigue. It will also help maintain your metabolism at a higher level, which is helpful if you're trying to lose weight or maintain a healthy weight. But as you know, too heavy a lunch can lead to right-after-lunch lethargy and fatigue. Eating a low-carb lunch lets you avoid the "down" feeling.

The Sandwich Struggle

The basic sandwich presents a problem for anyone trying to eat low carb. The problem, of course, is the bread. Some low-carb breads are available at grocery stores, but they certainly aren't offered in many restaurants, if any fast-food restaurants. If you choose to eat low-carb breads, be sure to check the carbohydrate count, it could still be higher than you'd like.

Our bread recipes in Chapter 22 are great if you want a sandwich and your carbohydrate allowance is on the high side at 45 carbs per meal or 135 carbs per day.

A little self-discipline goes a long way, too. Just think to say "Hold the bread," and you'll hardly notice its absence.

Salad to Go

Yield:	Serving size:	Prep time:	Cook time:
1 serving	2 cups	20 minutes	None

Each serving has:		
10 g carbohydrate	3 g fiber	7 g protein

Mixed greens	Seeds
Various vegetables	Salad dressings
Leftover meats	4-oz. portion cups
Cheese, grated or small cubes	Paper lunch bags
Nuts	

See suggestions that follow for a variety of ingredients to make these delicious salads.

1. Wash and dry all greens, and vegetables. In separate quart baggies, place $1\frac{1}{2}$ cups greens, squeeze out as much air as possible, and seal. In separate sandwich-size baggies, mix $\frac{1}{2}$ cup sliced or chopped vegetables, $\frac{1}{4}$ cup leftover meats, and a toppings combination including 1 tablespoon each cheese, nuts, or seeds.

2. Prepare favorite salad dressing recipes or select one from Chapter 20, and pour 2 to 4 tablespoons dressing into some small plastic containers.

3. In each paper lunch bag, place one of each various baggies and a salad dressing cup. Each lunch bag will contain greens, veggies, meat and/or cheese, nuts and seeds, as well as a portion of salad dressing or lemon juice.

4. Remember to pack a napkin, eating utensils, and salad bowl!

Ingredient suggestions:

Greens: Choose red leaf, green leaf, raw baby spinach, romaine, Bibb, shredded cabbage, or mixed greens in a bag that include arugula, radicchio, and dandelion.

Raw vegetables: Celery, peppers, cucumbers, carrots, mild onions, broccoli, cauliflower, yellow squash, mushrooms, snow peas, shelled soybeans, radishes, jicama, avocado, and cherry or grape tomatoes are simply delicious raw.

Canned vegetables: Other veggie choices are mushrooms, artichoke hearts, hearts of palm, asparagus, pearl onions, cut green beans, olives, chilies, and water chestnuts.

Meats: Leftover meats can be anything from last night's dinner or canned tuna, salmon, or chicken. Boiled eggs or leftover ham or sausage from breakfast can also be added to your salad.

Cheese: Any cheese cut into small bite-size cubes or grated, such as cheddar, Swiss, Parmesan, blue, or feta works well.

Nuts and seeds: These can include peanuts, macadamias, walnuts, almonds, pecans, pistachios, pine nuts, cashews, coconut, flaxseeds, or sesame seeds.

RECIPE FOR SUCCESS

Do you see that the world of salads is limited only by your own imagination and creative genius? If we omitted your favorite ingredient from this list, then by all means bag it for your next salad to go! You can substitute lemon juice for salad dressing.

Chicken Couscous

Yield:	Serving size:	Prep time:	Cook time:
6 servings	¾ cup	10 minutes	None
Each serving has:			
11 g carbohydrate	3 g fiber	15 g protein	

½ cup couscous

¾ cup boiling chicken broth

2 cups diced cooked chicken

2 large tomatoes, diced

¼ cup green onion, chopped

¼ cup radishes, sliced

½ cup cucumber, chopped

¼ cup olive oil

¼ cup lemon juice

¼ cup fresh parsley, snipped

¼ cup fresh mint leaves, minced, or 1 TB. dried mint

Salt and pepper to taste

Pine nuts or slivered almonds for garnish (optional)

1. Place couscous in a 2-quart casserole dish or bowl, and cover with boiling chicken broth; cover and let sit for 10 minutes until stock is absorbed.

2. In a medium bowl, combine chicken, tomatoes, green onion, radishes, and cucumber.

3. In a pint-size screw-top jar, combine olive oil, lemon juice, parsley, mint, salt, and pepper; shake well.

4. If couscous does not absorb all liquid, drain before adding dressing and chicken.

5. Pour olive oil dressing over couscous, fluff with fork, and mix in chicken and vegetable mixture. Sprinkle with nuts (if using) and serve.

RECIPE FOR SUCCESS

The flavors in this recipe mellow and blend together better if allowed to sit 30 minutes or longer. This dish is just as wonderful served cold and is a snap to make ahead of time for that special luncheon. Serve with Congealed Asparagus Salad and Parmesan Crackers (see recipe in Chapter 20), and you will still have plenty of room for scrumptious Chocolate Soufflé (see recipe in Chapter 25) for dessert.

Scotch Eggs

Yield:	Serving size:	Prep time:	Cook time:
6 servings	1 egg	20 minutes	30 minutes
Each serving has:			
3 g carbohydrate	1 g fiber	24 g protein	

2 TB. fresh parsley, chopped

¼ tsp. sage, optional

1 tsp. onion powder

1 lb. bulk sausage

6 hard-boiled eggs, peeled

2 large eggs, beaten

⅓ cup oat bran or ground oatmeal

¼ tsp. butter

1. Preheat the oven to 350°F.

2. Stir parsley, sage, and onion powder into sausage. Divide sausage into 6 even portions, and shape each into a 4-inch ball. Flatten and wrap around 1 peeled hard-boiled egg, covering egg completely.

3. Roll each sausage egg in beaten egg and then in oat bran. Bake on a buttered sheet pan for 30 minutes or until sausage is completely cooked.

4. Remove eggs from pan and serve. If making in advance, place cooled eggs in individual snack bags, and refrigerate up to 1 week.

TABLE TALK

Using scissors to snip fresh parsley and other twiggy herbs and spices is usually much easier than trying to chop. It's easy to snip a handful of green onions and keeps you from bruising the delicate foods.

Cold Cut Rollups

Yield:	Serving size:	Prep time:	Cook time:
6 servings	1 rollup	5 minutes	None
Each serving has:			
1 g carbohydrate	< 1 g fiber	14 g protein	

Lettuce leaves

½ lb. luncheon meat (ham, turkey, roast beef, or pastrami), sliced

½ lb. cheese (American, cheddar, Swiss, or provolone), thinly sliced

Mayonnaise

Mustard

Toothpicks

1. Place lettuce leaves on work space. Top with a slice each of meat and cheese.

2. Spread cheese with mayonnaise and mustard to taste. Roll up and secure with a toothpick.

Variation: Use fish or shellfish in place of luncheon meat. You can also use left-over sliced meat from dinner. Add sliced or cut-up vegetables such as cucumber, radishes, tomatoes, or green bell peppers.

RECIPE FOR SUCCESS

You can prepare rollups the night before and have them ready for a quick breakfast. Eat with an apple or other fruit, and you have a good breakfast. You can also pack these in a school lunch box. They are great with dill pickles as a condiment.

Egg Salad and Variations

Yield:	Serving size:	Prep time:	Cook time:
6 servings	1/2 cup	15 minutes	None

Each serving has:		
2 g carbohydrate	0 g fiber	13 g protein

12 hard-boiled and peeled eggs, chopped

1/2 tsp. salt

1/2 tsp. pepper

3 to 4 TB. mayonnaise

1. Combine eggs, salt, and pepper and mix to a paste with a fork. Add just enough mayonnaise to moisten. This makes basic egg salad. You can add any of the following variations to this mixture.

Variation 1: Add 1/2 cup chopped crisp-fried bacon.

Variation 2: Add 1/2 cup baby shrimp and 1/2 teaspoon curry powder.

Variation 3: Add 1/4 cup chopped pecans and 2 tablespoons flaxseeds.

Variation 4: Add 1/2 cup chopped ham, 1/2 teaspoon Dijon mustard, 1 tablespoon chopped fresh parsley, and 1/4 teaspoon chopped fresh dill.

Variation 5: Add 1/2 cup minced smoked salmon, 1 teaspoon minced onion, 1 tablespoon capers, and 1 tablespoon lemon juice.

Variation 6: Add sour cream to moisten rather than mayonnaise, 1 mashed anchovy, 1 teaspoon chopped chives, and 1 tablespoon chopped fresh cilantro.

Variation 7: Add 1 (3-ounce) can tuna, 1/4 teaspoon minced garlic, and 1/2 cup chopped celery.

Variation 8: Add 1/4 cup grated Parmesan or Asiago cheese.

RECIPE FOR SUCCESS

The possibilities for egg salad are endless and all appetizing. Here's one for every day of the week, but feel free to add in your own favorite meats, cheeses, and condiments.

Nut Butter Spreads

Yield:	Serving size:	Prep time:	Cook time:
1½ cups	2 tablespoons nut butter	15 minutes	None

Each serving has:		
0 g carbohydrate	0 g fiber	4 g protein

2 cups peanuts, almonds, pecans,
   macadamias, cashews, or
   filberts

1. Place nuts in a food processor or blender. Process until nut butter forms. You may need to scrape the side of the bowl several times to blend thoroughly.

2. Serve on vegetables, such as celery, jicama slices, carrot sticks, or cucumber slices.

3. You can also serve as a spread on fruit. Try bananas, peaches, melon, pears, apples, and oranges.

RECIPE FOR SUCCESS

Purchase nuts in bulk at the health food store or grocery warehouse to get the best prices. Nut butters are great for late-afternoon snacks. You can even eat the butters plain by the spoonful.

Mexican Layers with Veggies

Yield:	Serving size:	Prep time:	Cook time:
6 servings	½ cup	45 minutes plus time to chill	None

Each serving has:			
10 g carbohydrate	5 g fiber	15 g protein	

½ cup mayonnaise

½ cup fresh cilantro, chopped

¼ cup lime juice

1 tsp. cumin

½ tsp. black pepper

1 head lettuce, shredded

1 (15-oz.) can black beans, rinsed and drained

2 cups (8 oz.) cheddar cheese, shredded

1 large bell pepper, chopped

3 green onions, chopped

3 tomatoes, chopped

1. In a food processor, combine mayonnaise with cilantro, lime juice, cumin, and black pepper.

2. Either on a large platter or in a large glass bowl, layer ingredients in the following order: ½ lettuce, ⅓ mayonnaise mixture, ½ beans, cheese, bell pepper, onions, and tomatoes. Repeat layers and top with remaining mayonnaise mixture.

3. Cover and chill 1 to 2 hours.

RECIPE FOR SUCCESS

This is a meal in itself but has very little animal protein. You may slice boiled eggs on top or serve with one of the beefsteak recipes or the Beef and Pork Skewers (see recipe that follows). Cheese Apple Bake (see recipe in Chapter 15) make a great dessert, adding that additional serving of fruit to your day.

Beef and Pork Skewers

Yield:	Serving size:	Prep time:	Cook time:
12 servings	1 skewer	20 minutes	1½ hours

Each serving has:			
0 g carbohydrate	0 g fiber	16 g protein	

¾ lb. beef, cut into ½-in. cubes

¾ lb. pork, cut into ½-in. cubes

2 TB. butter

Salt and pepper to taste

1. Preheat the oven to 325°F.

2. Alternate beef and pork onto wooden 6-inch skewers. Place butter in a large skillet over medium-high heat. Add skewers and brown well. Sprinkle meat with salt and pepper.

3. Place meat skewers in an ovenproof dish. Cover meat with water. Cover the pan. Bake for 1 hour.

4. Eat like a chicken leg or remove meat from sticks. These can be eaten cold as well.

RECIPE FOR SUCCESS

Eat these warm when they come out of the oven and cold for lunches and breakfasts. They also make a great after-school or after-work snack. You can even take these along for a picnic lunch while hiking or bicycling.

The Least You Need to Know

- The new lunch box includes complete protein, fruit, vegetable, and an optional sweet treat.
- Try commercial low-carb breads or tortillas to reduce the carbs in a sandwich.
- Keep your refrigerator stocked with foods for lunch—such as cold cuts, hard-boiled eggs, leftovers, and cheese.
- Eating a low-carb lunch helps you avoid mid-afternoon energy letdown and fatigue.

Main Dish Entrées

The centerpiece of your dinner meals is a low-carb main dish made with delectable meats, poultry, fish, or seafood. The meat can be roasted, marinated, grilled, boiled, or even cooked in the oven in bags.

Appealing spices and aromas greet you as you sit down to enjoy these main dishes. The tastes are satisfying, whether savory or sweet, as they deliver high-quality complete protein to stoke your metabolism and give you tip-top nutrition.

Beef Dishes

In This Chapter

- Eating energizing meat
- Purchasing beef
- Planning meals with beef

Whatever form it comes in—steaks, roast beef, or hamburgers—beef is a favorite. It's hearty fare, real stick-to-your-ribs—but not fattening—kind of food and for good reason. The very intensity and rich taste of beef makes it ideal for eating low carb because, as you know, getting plenty of high-quality protein is a big factor in eating low carb and the focus of this chapter.

Beef gives that to you and more. By itself, it has no carbohydrates, yet it offers plenty of protein, vitamins, and minerals. Beef is filled with the highest concentration of B vitamins and trace minerals of any single food. It supplies ample amounts of the vitamin B_{12} that you can't get from vegetables alone. Oh, and it simply tastes good, too!

Get an Energy Lift

Beef is one of the perfect foods for staying energized all day long. It contains purines, which are a major component of nucleic acids. Nucleic acids are metabolized into energy more slowly than carbohydrates. Practically speaking, what does that mean? By eating beef you may be able to boost your metabolic burn rate and keep your energy level high through stressful and taxing situations. In short, beef is a great food for our busy lives.

You don't need to eat very much beef to stay energized. Typically, you only need 3 ounces cooked beef, which is about the size of a deck of cards. Yes, we have all been to restaurants that offer 16-ounce T-bone steaks or prime rib. Just think, you could eat five meals from that amount of beef! So avoid the mega-portions or share your entrée with a friend … or two or three!

Three ounces of cooked beef contain about 26 grams of high-quality, complete protein. A good formula for healthy adults is that you need about $\frac{1}{2}$ gram protein per day for each pound you weigh. A woman who weighs 150 pounds needs about 75 grams of protein a day. A man who weighs 200 pounds needs about 100 grams of protein a day. So even 3 ounces beef goes a long way to getting you the protein you need.

TABLE TALK

Four ounces raw meat yields about 3 ounces cooked—the weight listed in menus is always the precooked raw weight.

Beef for Your Body

If you have a heavy-duty day ahead of you, whether it's a day of business travel, hot and heavy negotiations, or hitting the ski slopes, go ahead and have some beef for breakfast. Your body will thank you.

While most of us won't cook up a feast for breakfast using the recipes here, they will make great breakfast from last night's dinner leftovers. You might also be surprised at how little time it takes to cook a small steak or meat patty for breakfast. Add some vegetables or fruit, and you are ready to roll into action.

TABLE TALK

Recent research indicates that eating lean beef combined with a lower-carbohydrate diet is excellent for weight loss. Of course, portion control is important, too. No matter how much you love beef, don't overeat. Three to five ounces is plenty.

Eating beef can also be good for your heart, but you'll definitely need to eat modest quantities. Be sure to cut off all the visible fat. That is saturated fat, and you don't need any extra. Choose lean cuts or cook slowly so the fat melts out of the meat and into the pot. Cooking in the slow cooker does this well, as does roasting or boiling the beef.

Beef-Jicama Chalupas

Yield:	Serving size:	Prep time:	Cook time:
6 servings	¾ cup	15 minutes	2 minutes
Each serving has:			
5 g carbohydrate	9 g fiber	19 g protein	

2 cups shredded cooked beef from Slow Cooker Pot Roast (see following recipe)	1 (4-oz.) can green chilies, diced
	½ cup cheddar or Monterey Jack cheese, shredded
1 cup commercial salsa	2 cups *jicama*, julienned
1 (8-oz.) can corn	2 tomatoes, diced

1. In a shallow, microwave-safe dish, mix beef, salsa, corn, and chilies. Heat on medium for about 1 minute, until warm. Top with cheese, and microwave until just melted.

2. Divide jicama onto 6 dinner plates. Spoon beef mixture on jicama, and top with diced tomatoes.

DEFINITION

Jicama is a root vegetable that originated in Mexico. It has a sweet crispness when eaten raw. It is low in sodium, has no fat, and is high in vitamin C. It adds crunch and freshness to salads and is great for a refreshing snack.

Slow Cooker Pot Roast

Yield:	Serving size:	Prep time:	Cook time:
16 servings	4 ounces	5 minutes	4 hours
Each serving has:			
0 g carbohydrate	0 g fiber	21 g protein	

3 lb. beef chuck roast	½ tsp. coarsely ground black pepper

1. Put beef into a slow cooker, season with pepper, and cover with the lid.

2. Turn on high and cook for 4 to 6 hours or until the meat is so tender that it can be cut with a fork.

Variation: This recipe is the easiest way to get cooked beef for tacos, barbecued beef, salads, and other recipes. Reheat or serve cold for lunches and snacks. You can vary the flavor each time you cook a roast by adding additional seasonings to the slow cooker. Suggestions include ¹⁄₂ cup beef broth or tomato sauce, onions, garlic, bell pepper, oregano, salsa, etc.

RECIPE FOR SUCCESS

The slow cooker is a great way to prepare a roast without slaving in the kitchen all day. The meat is moist and can be cut with a fork. Serve with plenty of vegetables. Use the pan drippings to make gravy, or serve with horseradish, chutney, or barbecue sauce.

Marinated London Broil

Yield:	Serving size:	Prep time:	Cook time:
6 servings	4 ounces	15 minutes plus marinating time	15 minutes

Each serving has:		
1 g carbohydrate	< 1 g fiber	26 g protein

1½ lb. flank steak

3 TB. red wine vinegar

1 clove garlic, minced

¼ tsp. crushed red pepper

2 TB. soy sauce

¼ cup olive oil

¼ tsp. coarsely ground black pepper

2 cups white mushrooms, sliced

2 TB. butter

1. Put steak, vinegar, garlic, crushed red pepper, soy sauce, olive oil, and black pepper into a resealable bag. *Marinate* for 2 to 4 hours or overnight in the refrigerator.

2. Cook on the grill or broil in the oven until done to taste, about 3 minutes on a side. At the same time, sauté mushrooms in butter in a heavy skillet until tender.

3. Slice meat very thin, and top with mushrooms.

Variation: Marvelous and economical, this recipe makes great leftovers for breakfast. You can also roll up pieces of fruit in the thin slices and send them to school with the kids. This steak is perfect for fajitas, chalupas, or topping your favorite green salad for lunch.

DEFINITION

Marinades are a blend of seasonings, oil, and acidic liquid. The acid in the marinade tenderizes meat and adds flavoring. Wine may be substituted for juice or vinegar in marinades; use white wine for a milder flavor for more delicate proteins such as fish or poultry. A red wine gives a stronger, more robust flavor and is usually used with red meat, game, and pork.

Sirloin with Lemon Sauce

Yield:	Serving size:	Prep time:	Cook time:
6 servings	4 ounces	15 minutes	15 minutes

Each serving has:		
1 g carbohydrate	< 1 g fiber	33 g protein

4 TB. butter

1 cup green onions, finely chopped

$\frac{1}{2}$ dried bay leaf

$\frac{1}{2}$ tsp. dried thyme

$1\frac{1}{2}$ cups dry red wine

$3\frac{1}{2}$ lb. boneless beef sirloin steak, about $1\frac{1}{2}$ in. thick

3 TB. fresh parsley, minced

1 TB. fresh lemon juice

1. In a large, heavy skillet, melt 2 tablespoons butter over high heat. Sauté onions, bay leaf, and thyme until onions are transparent, about 2 to 3 minutes. Add wine and cook until reduced by one-third.

2. Remove bay leaf, and pour sauce from the skillet and reserve. In the same skillet over high heat, sear steak for $1\frac{1}{2}$ minutes per side. Turn heat to medium, and let skillet cool slightly; add sauce, remaining 2 tablespoons butter, parsley, and lemon juice. Cook for an additional 2 to 4 minutes per side, depending on taste.

3. Cut steak into 2-inch diagonal strips, and serve with red wine sauce from skillet.

RECIPE FOR SUCCESS

Lemon adds lots of pizzazz to a dinner steak. Garnish with lemon twists. You can serve with rich or simple side dishes, such as creamed vegetables or a tossed vegetable salad.

Mustard Brisket

Yield:	Serving size:	Prep time:	Cook time:
12 servings	4 ounces	10 minutes	4 hours
Each serving has:			
2 g carbohydrate	0 g fiber	26 g protein	

1 (3-lb.) beef brisket, trimmed of excess fat	$\frac{1}{3}$ cup spicy mustard
2 cups water	1 tsp. cracked peppercorns
6 cloves garlic, peeled and sliced	1 tsp. dried tarragon
	$\frac{1}{4}$ cup green onions, chopped

1. Preheat the oven to 325°F.

2. Place brisket in a large baking pan. Add water to bottom of the baking pan. Cut slits all around brisket, and insert slices of garlic deep into meat.

3. In a small bowl, combine mustard, peppercorns, tarragon, and green onions. Rub mixture into brisket, covering well all over.

4. Cover the pan and bake for 4 hours or until meat is tender.

Beef Steak over Greens

Yield:	Serving size:	Prep time:	Cook time:
10 servings	4 ounces meat over 1 cup greens	15 minutes plus marinating overnight	20 minutes

Each serving has:			
4 g carbohydrate	1 g fiber	27 g protein	

¼ cup olive oil	2 TB. lemon juice
¼ cup Worcestershire sauce	1 TB. fresh parsley, chopped
1 tsp. garlic powder	Salt and pepper to taste
1 tsp. cayenne	6 cups mixed salad greens (red leaf, butter romaine, baby spinach, etc.)
1 (2-lb.) flank steak	3 TB. horseradish sauce
1 (8-oz.) pkg. sour cream	3 cucumbers, peeled and sliced
4 TB. prepared horseradish	

1. Combine olive oil, Worcestershire sauce, garlic powder, and cayenne in a gallon-size freezer bag. Add steak, seal bag, and refrigerate overnight. Turn the bag occasionally to spread marinade over all surfaces of steak.

2. In a pint jar with a screw-type lid, combine sour cream, prepared horseradish, lemon juice, parsley, salt, and pepper. Refrigerate until needed.

3. Heat the grill to medium-high heat. Remove steak from marinade, and throw away marinade. Place steak off direct heat, and close lid on grill; cook 8 to 10 minutes per side or until desired doneness. Let meat rest 10 to 15 minutes before cutting.

4. While meat is cooking, wash and dry salad greens, and tear into bite-size pieces. Toss with cucumber slices, and place 1 cup salad mix in individual bowls or on plates.

5. Cut steak into thin slices and place over greens. Drizzle with horseradish sauce and serve.

Variation: Grilled steak makes wonderful fajitas served over greens. Serve with Baked Onions (see recipe in Chapter 19). Pear Compote (see recipe in Chapter 21) makes the perfect ending to this satisfying meal. The leftover grilled steak makes delicious cold beef for breakfast or snacks, or bag up leftovers to add to tomorrow's mixed salad.

RECIPE FOR SUCCESS

This steak can just as easily be grilled, if desired. Serving with Vibrant Peppers and Tomatoes (see recipe in Chapter 19), Mock Mashed Potatoes (see recipe in Chapter 23), and Frosty Fruit (see recipe in Chapter 21) ensures the entire rainbow of colors and plenty of vitamins.

Rubbed Beef Steak

Yield:	Serving size:	Prep time:	Cook time:
10 servings	4 ounces	15 minutes plus marinating time	15 minutes

Each serving has:		
0 g carbohydrate	0 g fiber	27 g protein

1 (2-lb.) flank steak, pierced on all sides with fork	2 TB. paprika
1 TB. garlic powder	1 tsp. crushed red pepper
3 TB. oregano	1 tsp. salt
1 TB. black pepper	¼ cup dry mustard
	¼ tsp. olive oil

1. Place steak in a glass dish.

2. In a small bowl, blend garlic powder, oregano, black pepper, paprika, red pepper, salt, and dry mustard.

3. Spread rub onto all sides of flank steak, especially pushing into areas pierced with fork. Cover meat thoroughly, pressing rub onto meat. Cover the dish, and refrigerate for several hours or overnight.

4. Preheat the broiler. Oil the broiler pan, and place steak on the pan. Throw away any remaining seasoning from marinating raw meat. Set the pan 4 inches from the broiler unit, and broil on each side 5 minutes or until meat thermometer registers 145°F.

Beef with Vinaigrette Sauce

Yield:	Serving size:	Prep time:	Cook time:
6 servings	4 ounces with 2 tablespoons sauce	10 minutes	30 minutes

Each serving has:		
0 g carbohydrate	0 g fiber	32 g protein

1 (2-lb.) flank steak, grilled	1 tsp. black pepper
$\frac{1}{2}$ cup olive oil	$\frac{1}{2}$ tsp. crushed red pepper
2 TB. red wine vinegar or seasoned vinegar	1 tsp. dried rosemary or other herb of choice
2 cloves garlic, minced	

1. Slice cooked steak on the diagonal, against the grain, and arrange on a platter.

2. Combine olive oil, vinegar, garlic, black pepper, red pepper, and rosemary. Pour vinaigrette sauce over steak and serve.

Marinated Beef Kabobs

Yield:	Serving size:	Prep time:	Cook time:
6 servings	1 skewer	20 minutes plus marinating time	15 minutes

Each serving has:		
6 g carbohydrate	2 g fiber	33 g protein

2 TB. lemon or lime juice	2 large bell peppers, cut into $1\frac{1}{4}$-in. pieces
2 TB. olive oil	18 whole white mushrooms
2 tsp. sesame oil	12 grape or cherry tomatoes, leave whole
2 TB. water	
1 TB. spicy mustard	2 zucchini, cut into 1-in. slices
1 tsp. honey	2 large onions, cut into $1\frac{1}{4}$-in. pieces
1 tsp. basil	$\frac{1}{4}$ tsp. butter
1 tsp. crushed red pepper	
2 lb. boneless beef, cut into 1-in. cubes	

1. In a large bowl, combine lemon juice, olive oil, sesame oil, water, mustard, honey, basil, and red pepper; add beef, bell peppers, mushrooms, tomatoes, zucchini, and onions. Toss well and allow to marinate in refrigerator at least 2 hours or even overnight; turn occasionally.

2. Alternately thread beef and vegetables onto 6 long skewers.

3. Butter a broiler pan, and place kabobs on the pan 3 to 4 inches from heat. Broil 9 to 12 minutes for medium-rare to medium-done, turning occasionally to prevent overbrowning surface.

HOT POTATO

If using wooden skewers, be sure to soak them in water for 1 hour before using to prevent them from burning.

RECIPE FOR SUCCESS

If you prefer to grill, place kabobs over medium-hot coals and grill uncovered 8 to 11 minutes, turning occasionally. You may place beef and vegetables in a wire basket instead of threading onto skewers, if desired. For a fabulous next-day luncheon salad, double this recipe to have plenty of leftovers. Top a mixed green salad and sprinkle with sesame seeds and balsamic vinegar. Running late for work the next day? Grab a leftover skewer for a high-protein, high-vitamin breakfast!

Sautéed Steak with Green Peppercorns

Yield:	Serving size:	Prep time:	Cook time:
6 servings	½ steak, approximately 6 ounces	10 minutes plus 1 hour marinating time	20 minutes

Each serving has:			
0 g carbohydrate	0 g fiber	40 g protein	

2 TB. coarsely cracked green peppercorns

2 (1-lb.) steaks, ¾- to 1-in. thick

2 TB. butter

2 TB. olive oil

Salt and pepper to taste

½ cup beef stock, red wine, dry white wine, or vermouth

2 TB. softened butter

1. Press peppercorns onto both sides of meat. Place in a dish, cover, and refrigerate 1 hour.

2. Heat butter and oil in a heavy skillet over medium-high heat until butter foam begins to subside. With grease very hot but not burning, sauté steak on each side for 3 to 4 minutes. Steak will be medium-rare when a bit of red juice begins to ooze at surface.

3. Remove steak to a hot platter, and season to taste with salt and pepper. Keep warm while completing sauce.

4. Pour remaining oil and butter out of the skillet. Add stock and place the skillet over high heat. Scrape juices with a wooden spoon while rapidly boiling down liquid until it is reduced almost to syrup.

5. Remove from heat, and swirl softened butter into liquid until it is absorbed. Butter will thicken liquid into a light sauce.

6. Pour sauce over steak and serve.

RECIPE FOR SUCCESS

Steak with peppercorns seems to be a combination made in cook's heaven. The peppercorns add flavor and seem to make the steak more tender. Serve with at least one mildly seasoned side dish to prevent spice overload. Bland steamed peas, carrots, or broccoli would be great.

Beef Tandoor

Yield:	Serving size:	Prep time:	Cook time:
6 servings	¾ cup	15 minutes plus overnight marinating time	1½ hours

Each serving has:		
2 g carbohydrate	0 g fiber	30 g total protein

1 onion, coarsely chopped

3 cloves garlic, chopped

1 tsp. fresh ginger, minced

½ tsp. cumin

2 TB. coriander

1 TB. turmeric

¼ cup red pepper, chopped

¼ cup red wine vinegar

¼ cup olive oil

2 lb. beef stew meat

4 TB. butter

1. In a blender or food processor, process onion, garlic, ginger, cumin, coriander, turmeric, red pepper, red wine vinegar, and olive oil into thick marinade.

2. Thoroughly coat meat, and marinate in the refrigerator overnight.

3. In a heavy pot, brown meat in melted butter over high heat. Lower heat and simmer about 1 to $1^1/_2$ hours until tender. Stir occasionally.

Beef Stroganoff

Yield:	Serving size:	Prep time:	Cook time:
6 servings	$^1/_2$ cup	15 minutes	10 minutes
Each serving has:			
1 g carbohydrate	0 g fiber	32 g protein	

$1^1/_2$ lb. sirloin steak

6 TB. butter

$^1/_4$ onion, chopped

$^1/_2$ cup white mushrooms, sliced

$^1/_2$ tsp. salt

$^1/_2$ tsp. coarsely ground black pepper

1 TB. paprika

$^1/_2$ cup heavy cream

1. Cut meat into $^1/_2$- × 2-inch slices. Heat butter in a heavy pan. Sauté onion and mushrooms for about 3 minutes until tender. Add steak and cook for about 5 minutes or until tender. Season with salt, pepper, and paprika.

2. Slowly stir in cream. Heat without boiling. Serve at once. If you prefer, serve with Mock Mashed Potatoes (see recipe in Chapter 23).

Pot Roast with Caraway, Orange, and Ginger

Yield:	Serving size:	Prep time:	Cook time:
8 servings	4 ounces	30 minutes	5 to 7 hours
Each serving has:			
4 g carbohydrate	1 g fiber	32 g protein	

4 to 5 lb. boneless chuck roast or
    eye of round

4 TB. butter

2 medium onions, chopped

½ cup carrots, chopped

2 cups water

1 cup Burgundy wine

6 cloves garlic, crushed

1 bay leaf

2 TB. grated orange peel

1 TB. paprika

1 tsp. caraway seeds

1½ cups sour cream

2 TB. fresh or dried dill

2 TB. ginger

1. Preheat the oven to 275°F.

2. Heat roasting pan over medium-high heat, melt butter and brown roast on all sides. Remove roast from the pan, and sauté onions and carrots until tender. Add water, wine, garlic, bay leaf, orange peel, paprika, and caraway seeds to the pan. Heat to boiling and add roast.

3. Cover and bake for 5 to 7 hours or until tender.

4. Remove roast from the pan. Skim off fat. In the roasting pan, blend sour cream, dill, and ginger. Cook over low heat for 10 to 15 minutes. Don't boil.

5. Slice meat into thin slices and serve with sauce.

RECIPE FOR SUCCESS

This recipe, which has a Scandinavian flavor, is great for a winter fireside dinner.

Beef Fajitas

Yield:	Serving size:	Prep time:	Cook time:
6 servings	4 ounces beef with 3 tablespoons vegetables	15 minutes plus 2 to 3 hours marinating time	15 minutes

Each serving has:		
2 g carbohydrate	1 g fiber	32 g protein

¼ cup vinegar	1 medium onion, sliced
½ cup olive oil	1 green pepper, cut into strips
¼ cup lime juice	1 red pepper, cut into strips
1 clove garlic, mashed	2 TB. butter
¼ tsp. cumin	½ cup sour cream
¼ tsp. crushed red pepper	1 avocado, sliced (optional)
½ tsp. coriander	¾ cup salsa (optional)
1½ lb. flank steak	

1. Prepare marinade by combining vinegar, olive oil, lime juice, garlic, cumin, red pepper, and coriander in a resealable bag. Place beef in the bag, seal, and marinate 2 to 3 hours or overnight in the refrigerator.

2. When ready to cook, remove steak from the bag, saving marinade.

3. Boil marinade for 20 minutes before serving over meat, adding water if sauce gets too thick. Let simmer until ready to serve.

4. Slice steak into thin slices.

5. Sauté onion and red and green peppers in butter in a heavy skillet. Cook until crisp-tender. Remove to a side platter. Place steak slices in skillet and sauté steak until cooked through. Stir in marinade. Add onion and peppers.

6. Serve topped with sour cream, avocado, and salsa (if using). Guacamole and salsa may add more carbs to the scorecard.

 RECIPE FOR SUCCESS

Fajitas combine the best of south-of-the-border tastes with our American desire for meats and vegetables. Eat these fajitas with a fork instead of as tortillas, as they contain lots of carbohydrates.

Blue Cheese Rib Eyes

Yield:	Serving size:	Prep time:	Cook time:
8 servings	6 ounces	10 minutes	10 to 15 minutes

Each serving has:		
0 g carbohydrate	0 g fiber	21 g protein

2 lb. rib eye steaks	2 TB. olive oil
2 TB. butter	4 TB. blue cheese, crumbled

1. In a heavy skillet, heat butter and oil over medium-high heat. Place steak in skillet and cook until red juices appear on top of steak. Turn steak and cook 3–5 minutes more or until desired doneness. Turn off the stove. Divide blue cheese, and sprinkle over top of steaks. Let melt. Serve.

Garlic Roast

Yield:	Serving size:	Prep time:	Cook time:
6 servings	4 ounces	24 to 48 hours marinating time	6 hours

Each serving has:		
0 g carbohydrate	0 g fiber	32 g protein

1 (3- to 5-lb.) chuck roast	¼ tsp. salt
4 to 6 cloves garlic, cut into slivers	¼ tsp. pepper
1 cup red wine vinegar	3 TB. olive oil
1 TB. garlic powder	2 cups strong coffee
1 TB. onion powder	2 cups water

1. Pierce meat and insert slivered garlic cloves all over roast. Place meat in a heavy plastic bag, pour vinegar over meat, and sprinkle with garlic powder, onion powder, salt, and pepper. Cover and refrigerate for 24 to 48 hours. Turn every 12 hours.

2. Preheat the oven to 225°F.

3. Place oil in a heavy pan, and heat over medium heat. Add roast and brown on all sides. Pour coffee and water over meat, cover, and place in oven; bake for 4 to 6 hours until meat is tender and easily pierced by a knife point.

TABLE TALK

Adding the coffee to the pot roast helps tenderize the meat because coffee is acidic. It also lends a warm earthy aroma and flavor to the beef.

RECIPE FOR SUCCESS

Serve this tender roast with Southern Greens (see recipe in Chapter 19), Tasty Turnips (see recipe in Chapter 19), and Marinated Tomato Slices (see recipe in Chapter 20). But remember to save room for a slice of Chocolate Amaretto Cheesecake (see recipe in Chapter 25).

Stuffed Steak

Yield:	Serving size:	Prep time:	Cook time:
1 steak	6 ounces steak	30 minutes	60 minutes
Each serving steak has without stuffing:			
0 g carbohydrate	0 g fiber	42 g protein	

6 oz. boneless top sirloin steak, cut 1½ to 2 in. thick

Worcestershire sauce diluted in water or red wine for basting

Stuffing of choice (see suggestions that follow)

1. Preheat the oven to 350°F or grill, depending on cooking method desired.

2. Cut slit through center of steak to within ½ inch of edge. This will form a pocket to hold stuffing.

3. To grill steak, heat coals to medium-hot and place steak to the side to smoke for about 20 minutes, turning frequently until desired doneness. If needed, brush with Worcestershire sauce or red wine to keep moist.

4. To bake steak, place steak in a buttered roasting pan; add $\frac{1}{2}$ cup water to pan, and sprinkle steak with a few tablespoons Worcestershire sauce or red wine. Bake 1 hour or until desired doneness.

Choose from the following stuffings:

Pecan Stuffing

Pecan Stuffing has:		
9 g carbohydrate	0 g fiber	4 g protein

$\frac{1}{2}$ cup pecans (may substitute any nut)

2 TB. apple or orange juice

$\frac{1}{2}$ cup parsley leaves

$1\frac{1}{4}$ cups fresh fruit (apples, pears, etc.)

$\frac{1}{4}$ cup dried fruit (cranberries, apricots, raisins, etc.)

1. Combine pecans, juice, parsley, fresh fruit, and dried fruit in a food processor. Chop the ingredients by pulsing the processor.

Pesto Stuffing

Pesto Stuffing has:		
4 g carbohydrate	0 g fiber	9 g protein

$1\frac{1}{2}$ cups fresh basil leaves (for milder flavor substitute parsley)

2 cloves garlic

$\frac{1}{4}$ cup pine nuts (may substitute any nut)

$\frac{3}{4}$ cup fresh Parmesan cheese, grated

$\frac{1}{2}$ cup olive oil

1. Process basil, garlic, and nuts into thick paste; add cheese and process until very thick. Slowly add oil and continue to process until combined well.

Roasted Pepper Pesto Stuffing

Roasted Pepper Stuffing has:

4 g net carbohydrate   0 g fiber   2 g protein

¼ cup pesto from Pesto Stuffing
(recipe earlier in this chapter)

1 (7-oz.) jar roasted red pepper (or
substitute pimiento or dried
tomatoes)

2 TB. garlic, minced

1. Combine pesto, red pepper, and garlic well.

 RECIPE FOR SUCCESS

You can always try a stuffing of your own choosing. Simply combine your favorite
herbs and one vegetable or fruit with 2 tablespoons of liquid (if ingredients
appear dry).

The Least You Need to Know

- Beef gives you energy with high concentrations of B vitamins and trace
  elements.
- Eating beef works for fat-restricted diets as well as low-carb.
- Beef works well with other strong flavors.
- Add vegetable and/or fruit side dishes to your beef main course meals.

Ground Meat Dishes

In This Chapter

- Versatility of ground meat
- Making everyday food
- Choosing your fat content

Start with a pound of ground meat, and you can seemingly do almost anything, at least as far as a good meal is concerned. Ground meat is versatile and blends comfortably with many flavors, such as Italian, German, Greek, Mexican, Asian, and good old American.

Ground meat main-course dishes are usually easy to make and easy to serve. While most of us think of ground meat as something reserved for family dinners, you can proudly take several of the recipes in this chapter, such as lasagna and meatloaf, to potluck dinners or serve them to company.

Ground meat by itself has no carbohydrates. In these recipes, the carbohydrates come from other ingredients that add flavor, texture, and taste. Beef, pork, veal, and turkey are the most common types of ground meat.

We suggest you always keep a couple pounds ground meat in the freezer, so you'll always have some high-quality complete protein on hand for dinner. You can defrost it quickly in the microwave and have it ready to cook within 6 minutes.

To quickly defrost one pound ground meat in the microwave, set power level to defrost. Place meat, uncovered, on a microwave dish or tray. Defrost for 3 minutes. Scrape off softened meat and set aside. Break up remaining block and microwave on defrost for 2 to 3 more minutes.

Cooking Ground Meat

Not all ground beef is the same. It comes prepackaged with varying amounts of fat. The amounts range from 20 percent all the way down to 4 percent. The fat percentage you choose depends on your personal taste preference. Factors to consider when making your choice include (1) how you are going to cook the beef, (2) if you like the taste of fat in your food, and (3) what your personal dietary restrictions are. If you need to eat lower fat, then go for the lower percentages of fat in your ground beef.

Ground turkey ranges between 7 to 15 percent fat, so don't be fooled by thinking that if it's turkey, it has to be low fat. Ground pork is about 15 percent. Sausage is higher at about 25 percent.

When ground meat is cooked, whether browned for a dish like spaghetti, or baked as for a meatloaf, much of the fat is cooked out. This is called shrinkage. The fattier ground meats shrink down to less volume as the fat cooks out. Draining the fat from the meat leaves far less fat in the food. So let taste be the deciding factor in purchasing ground meat.

Hamburger with Mushrooms and Cream

Yield:	Serving size:	Prep time:	Cook time:
6 servings	½ cup	15 minutes	15 minutes
Each serving has:			
3 g carbohydrate	1 g fiber	9 g protein	

1 lb. ground beef	1 tsp. tarragon
½ cup onions, minced	1 cup white mushrooms, sliced
1 tsp. salt	1 cup heavy cream
¼ tsp. ground pepper	1 cup sour cream

1. Brown ground beef and onions together; drain off excess fat.

2. Add salt, pepper, tarragon, and mushrooms. Cook 5 minutes. Add heavy cream, simmer uncovered for 10 minutes, and stir in sour cream.

Picadille Dip

Yield:	Serving size:	Prep time:	Cook time:
8 servings	½ cup	20 minutes	30 minutes

Each serving has:		
8 g carbohydrate	3 g fiber	32 g protein

1 lb. ground pork sausage, your choice of flavor

1 lb. ground beef

4 green onions, chopped

1 tsp. cumin

1 cup toasted slivered almonds

1 tsp. dried oregano

1 tsp. garlic salt

½ tsp. black pepper

½ TB. sugar

1 cup pimiento, diced

1 (8-oz.) can tomatoes with jalapeños

2 (8-oz.) cans tomato sauce

1. Cook and drain sausage and beef. Add onions, cumin, almonds, oregano, garlic salt, pepper, sugar, pimiento, tomatoes with jalapeños, and tomato sauce; simmer 30 minutes.

2. Serve warm.

RECIPE FOR SUCCESS

You can serve Picadille Dip in small soup bowls and eat with a spoon or serve it with vegetable scoops, such as celery, jicama, and zucchini. Put over a bed of shredded jicama for eating as an open-face taco. You can even serve it over spaghetti squash as a main dish.

Fruit-Stuffed Meat Loaf

Yield:	Serving size:	Prep time:	Cook time:
6 servings	1 slice	30 minutes	1½ hours

Each serving has:		
14 g carbohydrate	2 g fiber	32 g protein

1½ lb. ground beef chuck

½ lb. ground lean pork

2 large eggs, lightly beaten

½ cup breadcrumbs

1½ tsp. salt

¼ tsp. black pepper

¼ cup raisins

¼ cup dried apricots, chopped

¼ cup fresh parsley, chopped

½ cup onion, chopped

½ tsp. sage

¼ tsp. dried thyme

½ cup beef broth

1. Preheat the oven to 350°F.

2. Combine beef, pork, eggs, breadcrumbs, salt, and pepper in a bowl and mix well. On a large piece of heavy-duty aluminum foil, spread mixture in a rectangle about ½-inch thick.

3. Combine raisins, apricots, parsley, onion, sage, thyme, and beef broth; mix thoroughly. Spread over meat loaf mixture and then roll up meat and filling like a jellyroll. Bring the foil up around the roll, and fold over to seal.

4. Place the package on a foil-lined baking sheet, and bake 1 hour. Open the foil to allow surface to brown, and bake 30 minutes longer. Let cool 5 minutes, and slice into 6 servings.

RECIPE FOR SUCCESS

Meat loaf is so versatile! Use it for a hot meal, serve it cold for lunches and breakfasts. Have a late-afternoon snack with a half-slice. It definitely will tide you over until a late dinner. This meat loaf has extra flair with the fruit stuffing.

Wild Rice and Beef Casserole

Yield:	Serving size:	Prep time:	Cook time:
6 servings	¾ cup	40 minutes	1 hour

Each serving has:			
10 g carbohydrate	< 1 g fiber	30 g protein	

4 cups boiling water	1 TB. soy sauce
¾ cup wild rice	½ tsp. curry powder
1 lb. ground beef	½ cup butter (1 stick)
3 cups chicken broth	⅓ cup onion, finely chopped
1½ tsp. salt	1 lb. white mushrooms, sliced
1 bay leaf	½ lb. sharp cheddar cheese, grated

1. Preheat the oven to 350°F.

2. Pour boiling water over rice, and let stand 15 minutes. Meanwhile, brown beef in a skillet and drain.

3. Drain rice; add broth, salt, bay leaf, soy sauce, and curry powder to rice.

4. Melt butter in a heavy skillet, add onion, and sauté until tender. Add mushrooms and sauté 3 minutes. Add browned beef, and stir over medium heat for about 5 minutes.

5. Combine rice mixture with meat mixture in a 9 × 14-inch casserole dish. Top with cheese, and bake 1 hour. Remove bay leaf before serving.

 RECIPE FOR SUCCESS

Wild rice has a strong enough flavor to enhance the beef in this recipe. This dish has a higher carb count than other beef recipes, so serve it with very low-carb vegetable dishes such as steamed vegetables and a tossed salad.

Eggplant with Ground Beef

Yield:	Serving size:	Prep time:	Cook time:
6 servings	½ cup	15 minutes	1 hour
Each serving has:			
7 g carbohydrate	2 g fiber	20 g protein	

1 large eggplant, peeled and diced

1 lb. lean ground beef

1 large onion, chopped

1 large bell pepper, chopped

1 stalk celery, diced

1 clove garlic, minced

1 (15-oz.) can diced tomatoes, drained and juice reserved

½ cup liquid from tomatoes

1 TB. tomato paste

Salt and black pepper to taste

1 cup shredded cheddar cheese

1. Preheat the oven to 350°F.

2. In a medium pot bring 6 cups of water to a boil and boil eggplant for 5 minutes. Set aside.

3. In a large skillet, brown beef and drain. Add onion, bell pepper, celery, and garlic to meat in the skillet; sauté 10 minutes or until onions are clear. Add drained tomatoes, ½ cup liquid from tomatoes, tomato paste, salt, pepper, and eggplant; simmer 30 minutes covered.

4. Pour mixture into a buttered casserole dish and top with grated cheese. Bake 20 minutes.

RECIPE FOR SUCCESS

This is an easy dish to serve after a long, busy day. Any leftovers will freeze well for a quick lunch another day. Pair this casserole with fresh Cranberry Salad (see recipe in Chapter 20) and steamed broccoli.

TABLE TALK

Plan ahead when using the food processor to chop fresh seasoning vegetables. It's easy to put in an extra onion or bell pepper, etc. Package your chopped veggies in amounts you usually need for sautéing, and freeze in small freezer bags. This makes cooking a breeze when needing a few veggies to sauté for a dish. Rule of thumb is one chopped medium onion or bell pepper is equal to about ½ cup each. Of course, you do not have to be exact with seasoning vegetables as you cook to your family's taste preferences.

Portobello Pizzas

Yield:	Serving size:	Prep time:	Cook time:
6 servings	2 mushroom pizzas	20 minutes	10 minutes

Each serving has:		
7 g carbohydrate	2 g fiber	17 g protein

½ lb. ground beef

1 small onion, diced

12 (5- to 6-in.) portobello mushrooms

2½ TB. olive oil

¼ cup freshly grated Parmesan cheese

6 (¼-in.) slices tomato

1 tsp. oregano

1 tsp. black pepper

1 cup shredded mozzarella cheese

1. Preheat the oven to 375°F.

2. Crumble and brown beef in a skillet with diced onions; drain and keep warm.

3. Clean mushrooms by wiping with a damp paper towel. In a large skillet, warm 2 tablespoons olive oil; add mushrooms and brown on both sides.

4. Place mushrooms on a baking sheet oiled with ½ tablespoon olive oil. Cover with Parmesan cheese, and add ground beef. Place 1 tomato slice on each mushroom, top with oregano and pepper, and sprinkle with mozzarella cheese.

5. Bake for 10 minutes.

RECIPE FOR SUCCESS

These mini pizzas use the portobello mushrooms for a base. They are wonderful appetizers as well as being highlighted as the main dish. Serve with basmati rice pilaf, Green Bean Almandine (see recipe in Chapter 19), and mixed fresh fruit.

HOT POTATO

Never store mushrooms in plastic bags. Refrigerate in containers that allow air to circulate around each mushroom, as moisture will cause mushrooms to deteriorate quickly.

Chili Meat Loaf

Yield:	Serving size:	Prep time:	Cook time:
10 servings	1 (½-inch) slice	30 minutes	50 minutes

Each serving has:		
7 g carbohydrate	2 g fiber	33 g protein

2 TB. butter	2 tsp. cumin
1 medium onion, diced	4 medium tomatoes, diced
1 red bell pepper, diced	1 lb. ground beef
2 tsp. garlic, minced	½ lb. ground sausage
2 fresh jalapeño peppers, diced	2 large eggs, lightly beaten
2 TB. chili powder	1 cup frozen corn kernels
2 tsp. salt	1 cup sharp cheddar cheese, shredded
2 tsp. oregano	

1. Preheat the oven to 350°F.

2. In a large skillet, heat butter and sauté onion, bell pepper, garlic, jalapeños, chili powder, salt, oregano, and cumin. Cover and cook, stirring occasionally, until vegetables are soft, about 10 minutes. Add tomatoes and cook another 10 minutes. Remove from heat to cool.

3. Combine ground beef and sausage. Add cooked mixture plus eggs and corn. Press into two 9 × 5-in. loaf pans.

4. Bake 50 minutes. Pour off any pan juices. Sprinkle cheese over loaves, and return to the oven until cheese melts. Cool 5 minutes, and cut each loaf into 5 slices to serve.

RECIPE FOR SUCCESS

This recipe is a tangy alternative to meat loaf. Serve with salsa and guacamole salad. Leftovers are great for lunches and breakfasts.

Stuffed Green Peppers

Yield:	Serving size:	Prep time:	Cook time:
4 servings	1 stuffed pepper	20 minutes	30 minutes

Each serving has:		
7 g carbohydrate	3 g fiber	34 g protein

4 green peppers	1 lb. ground beef
Boiling water	2 large eggs, lightly beaten
2 slices bacon, diced	Salt and pepper to taste
2 TB. butter	¼ tsp. dried parsley
1 small onion, diced	¼ tsp. dried basil
¾ cup celery, chopped	

1. Preheat the oven to 350°F.

2. Cut a slice from top of each pepper, and remove seeds and membrane. Cook pepper shells in boiling water for 5 minutes. Drain well.

3. In a heavy skillet, cook bacon until crisp. Remove bacon and add butter, onion, and celery, and sauté until tender. Remove mixture and set aside. Brown and drain ground beef. Add vegetable mixture back into the skillet, and set off heat. Stir in eggs, salt, pepper, parsley, and basil.

4. Fill pepper shells with meat mixture, and place in a greased baking dish. Pour hot water to a depth of ¼ inch around peppers. Bake 30 minutes.

 RECIPE FOR SUCCESS

The green peppers in this recipe make a tidy package for the seasoned ground beef mixture. Plus the peppers add additional flavor. Serve with one more vegetable and a light mousse or fruit soufflé for dessert.

Cabbage Rolls

Yield:	Serving size:	Prep time:	Cook time:
6 servings	2 rolls	20 minutes	1 hour

Each serving has:			
8 g carbohydrate	2 g fiber	10 g protein	

1 large head cabbage	2 TB. Worcestershire sauce
1 lb. ground meat	1 tsp. lemon juice
1 medium onion, diced	Salt and pepper to taste
1 large egg	1 cup water
½ tsp. cinnamon	1 (8-oz.) can tomato sauce
1 (6-oz.) can tomato paste	1 bell pepper, sliced

1. Preheat the oven to 350°F.

2. Remove 12 large leaves from cabbage, and parboil until softened. Trim off thick portion of each leaf.

3. In a bowl, mix together meat, diced onion, egg, cinnamon, tomato paste, Worcestershire sauce, lemon juice, salt, and pepper.

4. Line the bottom of a baking dish with extra cabbage leaves, and cover with water.

5. Place mound of meat mixture on each cabbage leaf, roll up, and place seam side down in the cabbage-lined dish. Pour on tomato sauce, and top with green pepper slices.

6. Cover the pan, and bake 1 hour.

RECIPE FOR SUCCESS

This meat stuffing is wonderful in hollowed out zucchini or eggplant boats. Serve with Curried Fruit on Skewers (see recipe in Chapter 21).

Spaghetti Sauce

Yield:	Serving size:	Prep time:	Cook time:
6 servings	¾ cup	25 minutes	1 hour

Each serving has:		
7 g carbohydrate	2 g fiber	14 g protein

1 onion, chopped	¼ cup green olives, sliced
½ cup sliced white mushrooms	½ tsp. fennel seeds
1 tsp. garlic, minced	1 tsp. salt
2 TB. butter	½ tsp. black pepper
1 lb. ground beef	2 TB. tomato paste
1 tsp. dried oregano	1 (28-oz.) can whole tomatoes
¼ cup black olives, sliced	

1. In a large heavy pot, sauté onion, mushrooms, and garlic in butter until tender. Remove from pan and set aside. Place ground beef in the pan and brown; drain. Return onion mixture to the pan, and add oregano, black and green olives, fennel seeds, salt, pepper, and tomato paste. Cut whole tomatoes into quarters, and add to the pot. Blend thoroughly.

2. Simmer for 1 hour, stirring occasionally. Add water if sauce looks too thick.

Variation: If you're in a rush to prepare the spaghetti sauce, try this: Brown 1 pound ground beef in a heavy skillet. Add 1 large container commercially prepared spaghetti sauce. Then add more of the seasonings you like—onion salt, minced garlic, crushed red pepper, fennel seed, oregano, and whatever else sounds good to you. Continue to cook a couple minutes and serve.

RECIPE FOR SUCCESS

Everyone loves spaghetti. You can double this or even triple it to feed a crowd. Serve it over cooked spaghetti squash. You can spoon sauce into half a squash for each serving, or remove the spaghetti-type fibers first from the squash shells.

Tamale Pie

Yield:	Serving size:	Prep time:	Cook time:
6 servings	¾ cup	30 minutes	50 minutes

Each serving has:		
19 g carbohydrate	4 g fiber	11 g protein

1 lb. lean ground beef	2 TB. chili powder
1 large onion, chopped	Salt and black pepper to taste
1 green bell pepper, chopped	1 (15-oz.) can kidney beans, drained
1 jalapeño pepper, diced (optional)	1 cup frozen whole-kernel corn
2 TB. taco seasoning	2 (8-oz.) cans tomato sauce
1 tsp. garlic, minced	

1. Preheat the oven to 400°F.

2. In a large skillet, brown ground beef. Drain off excess fat. Combine meat, onion, green pepper, jalapeño (if using), taco seasoning, garlic, chili powder, salt, and black pepper. Cook over medium heat until tender.

3. Using a 9 × 9-inch glass baking dish, place a layer of meat sauce on the bottom. Then layer with kidney beans. Add more meat sauce; top layer with corn; and add remaining meat mixture. Pour tomato sauce over all.

4. Bake for 20 minutes.

RECIPE FOR SUCCESS

This pie uses no crust, but the layering makes for a festive presentation. Serve it with shredded cheddar cheese, salsa, and guacamole or avocado salad.

HOT POTATO

This tamale pie contains 19 grams net carbs per serving, so it may seem too high to you. But it contains a meal's worth of vegetables plus healthy fiber and carbs from the kidney beans. Even if you're planning to eat only 25 grams of carbohydrates per meal, this recipe is a winner.

Lasagna

Yield:	Serving size:	Prep time:	Cook time:
8 servings	1 section	20 minutes	45 minutes plus standing time

Each serving has:			
6 g carbohydrate	< 1 g fiber	17 g protein	

1 lb. ground beef	$\frac{1}{2}$ cup Parmesan cheese, grated
1 (15-oz.) can tomato sauce	1 large egg
1 garlic clove, minced	$1\frac{1}{2}$ lb. zucchini, cut lengthwise into $\frac{1}{4}$-in. thick slices
1 tsp. dried basil	
2 tsp. dried rosemary, crumbled	1 cup mozzarella cheese, shredded
$1\frac{1}{2}$ cups ricotta cheese	

1. Preheat the oven to 350°F.

2. Brown ground beef in a large skillet and drain. Stir in tomato sauce, garlic, basil, and rosemary. Heat to boiling. Reduce heat and simmer about 10 minutes.

3. Mix ricotta, $\frac{1}{4}$ cup Parmesan, and egg in a small bowl.

4. In 9 × 13-inch greased baking pan, layer zucchini, cheese mixture, meat sauce, and mozzarella. Repeat. Sprinkle remaining $\frac{1}{4}$ cup grated Parmesan on top.

5. Bake for 45 minutes. Let stand 20 minutes before serving. Slice into 8 servings.

RECIPE FOR SUCCESS

Don't let the zucchini intimidate you. It takes on the wonderful Italian aromatic flavors of the lasagna and provides a great low-carb way to layer the cheeses and meat. Plus, the zucchini adds another healthful vegetable to the meal.

Chinese Meatballs

Yield:	Serving size:	Prep time:	Cook time:
6 servings	12 meatballs	20 minutes	40 minutes

Each serving has:		
7 g carbohydrate	6 g fiber	29 g protein

Each ¼ cup sauce serving has:		
13 g carbohydrate	0 g carbs	< 1 g protein

1 TB. soy sauce

1½ lb. ground beef

¼ cup celery, minced

¼ cup water chestnuts, minced

2 cloves garlic, minced

½ cup oat bran or ground oatmeal

2 large eggs, beaten

For Sauce:

1 cup tomato juice

1 TB. molasses

½ cup apple cider vinegar

2 TB. cornstarch

2 TB. soy sauce

½ cup pineapple juice

½ cup pineapple tidbits

½ green pepper, cut into strips

1. Preheat the oven to 350°F.

2. Mix 1 tablespoon soy sauce with ground beef, celery, water chestnuts, garlic, oat bran, and eggs. Form into 72 (1-inch) balls. Bake in a large roasting pan or lipped cookie sheet for 30 minutes.

3. For sauce, combine tomato juice, molasses, vinegar, cornstarch, 1 tablespoon soy sauce, pineapple juice, pineapple tidbits, and green pepper. Cook for 3 minutes or until slightly thickened. Add meatballs and simmer for 10 minutes. Remove meatballs from sauce, and serve alone for fewer carbohydrates.

RECIPE FOR SUCCESS

As a main dish with an Asian flair, serve with Ginger Carrots (see recipe in Chapter 19) and Mandarin Orange Spinach (see recipe in Chapter 20). Make the meatballs miniature-size, and serve with the warm sauce over fresh baby spinach for a delicious sweet-and-sour wilted salad; garnish with slivered almonds.

HOT POTATO

Eat the sauce in this recipe sparingly to avoid overloading on carbs. Have some, but not too much, so you can enjoy the taste, and comfortably stick with your eating plan.

Italian Meatballs

Yield:	Serving size:	Prep time:	Cook time:
6 servings	12 meatballs	20 minutes	30 minutes
Each serving has:			
1 g carbohydrate	6 g fiber	35 g protein	

1½ lb. ground beef

2 large eggs, beaten

½ cup oat bran or ground oatmeal

¼ cup onion, minced

3 cloves garlic, minced

½ tsp. dried oregano

¼ tsp. dried basil

¼ tsp. dried marjoram

¼ tsp. crushed red pepper

1. Preheat the oven to 350°F.

2. Combine beef, eggs, oat bran, onion, garlic, oregano, basil, marjoram, and red pepper. Form into 72 (1-inch) meatballs. Bake for 30 minutes in a large roasting pan or lipped cookie sheet.

3. Serve meatballs in your favorite Italian sauce over Vegetable Pasta (see recipe in Chapter 22) or Egg Pancake (see recipe in Chapter 4). Also, roll up the meatballs in large romaine leaves to make a delicious finger food!

TABLE TALK

For convenience, you may substitute Italian seasoning mix for the individual herb combination in this recipe.

The Least You Need to Know

- The versatility and convenience of ground meat lets you create interesting low-carb main courses.
- Use the ground meat—beef, sausage, turkey, or pork—that appeals to you in these recipes.
- Keep ground meat as a staple in your freezer for quick meals.
- Purchase ground meat with the fat percentage that meets your taste and dietary requirements.

Pork, Ham, and Veal Dishes

In This Chapter

- Cooking with pork
- Choosing pork and veal for meals
- Recognizing many cuts and choices

For many of us, just the smell of bacon cooking on a Saturday morning mesmerizes us enough to make us roll out of bed and stumble into the kitchen for breakfast. The aroma is irresistible. The enticing smell of pork ribs on the grill or Grandma's baked ham for holidays and special occasions elicits the same ardor.

The truth is, we love ham, bacon, and ribs. We love pork. It tastes good, and now we know it is also good for us. Pork contains plenty of essential amino acids to stoke metabolism. Plus, it's a cook's delight. The recipes in this chapter highlight pork's ability to blend well with many other foods and to be enhanced with many different spices and herbs. And best of all, pork has no carbs and is ideal for a low-carb eating plan.

Myths and Half-Truths

Pork has been subject to bad media spin for hundreds of years. So let's clear the air on the truth about pork.

Pork definitely has fat, as does any other meat. Through roasting and grilling the fattier cuts, such as ribs and ham, some of the fat is rendered out of the meat. The cooked pork you eat contains far less fat than it did before cooking.

Pork loin and pork chops often have very little to no marbling of fat and, so, contain less fat, even before cooking. Trimming the visible fat from such cuts either before or after cooking helps reduce your fat intake even further.

Part of pork's bad rep comes from earlier methods used to raise pigs that resulted in uncooked pork containing a dangerous parasitic roundworm which causes trichinosis. But a recent report from the USDA states that only 1 in 1,000 pigs are now found to contain the trichinosis-causing parasite. But just in case, never eat raw or partially cooked pork. Cooking the meat to an internal temperature of 137°F kills the parasite. To be safe, pork needs to be cooked to an internal temperature of 160°F. The cooked meat must be white or grayish throughout, without a trace of pink. When pricked with a fork, the juices must run clear and not be slightly pink.

HOT POTATO

When handling all raw meats and fish, and especially chicken and pork, be sure to wash all utensils and cutting boards thoroughly in hot soapy water to avoid contamination and prevent disease.

Tenderizing the White Meats

The light cuts of pork, such as tenderloin and chops, can turn out tough and chewy because these cuts have virtually no fat marbling and tight muscle fibers. However, marinades can solve the problem. Marinades contain an acidic liquid, usually vinegar, alcohol, or soy sauce, that helps break down the tight muscle fibers and makes the meat more tender and easier to chew. Some of the ingredients in our recipes also serve to tenderize the meat, such as sauerkraut, apples, and wine.

Veal is also a light meat that has relatively little fat and very tight muscle fibers. We can use two preparation methods to make the veal tender. First, we can pound thin slices of veal with a meat hammer to break up the muscle tissue. Pounding makes the meat quite thin. The second way to tenderize veal is by marinating.

Country Pâté

Yield:	Serving size:	Prep time:	Cook time:
25 servings	1 ($\frac{1}{2}$-inch) slice	$1\frac{1}{2}$ hours	$1\frac{1}{2}$ hours

Each serving has:		
1 g carbohydrate	< 1 g fiber	13 g protein

$\frac{3}{4}$ lb. bacon

1 TB. butter

1 onion, chopped

1 lb. pork, ground

$\frac{1}{2}$ lb. veal, finely chopped

$\frac{1}{2}$ lb. chicken livers, finely chopped

$\frac{1}{2}$ cup pistachios, shelled

2 cloves garlic, crushed

$\frac{1}{2}$ tsp. ground allspice

Pinch ground cloves

Pinch ground nutmeg

2 small eggs, lightly beaten

$\frac{1}{2}$ cup heavy cream

Salt and pepper to taste

$\frac{1}{2}$ lb. ham, cut in thin strips

1 bay leaf

25 Bibb or Romaine lettuce leaves

25 dill pickle slices

1. Preheat the oven to 350°F.

2. Line a 2-quart baking dish with a lid with bacon, reserving a few slices for the top.

3. Melt butter in a small pan, and sauté onion until soft but not brown. Combine with pork, veal, chicken livers, pistachios, garlic, allspice, cloves, nutmeg, eggs, heavy cream, salt, and pepper. Check seasoning. It should have a generous amount of salt and pepper.

4. Spread $\frac{1}{3}$ mixture in the baking dish. Layer with half ham strips and repeat.

5. Cover with last third of meat mixture. Lay remaining slices of bacon on top, then top with bay leaf. Place lid on baking dish.

6. Set the baking dish in a shallow roasting pan filled with 2 to 3 inches hot water. Bake $1\frac{1}{2}$ hours. Remove bay leaf.

7. Cool pâté until it is tepid before removing lid. Refrigerate 3 days or up to a week before serving.

8. As a first course, slice and serve on lettuce leaves, such as romaine or Bibb, with small dill pickles.

RECIPE FOR SUCCESS

Pâté is wonderful for low-carb eating. This pâté is great for meals, appetizers, and snacks. The combination of meats is very European.

Pork Chops and Cabbage

Yield:	Serving size:	Prep time:	Cook time:
8 servings	1 pork chop and 1 cup vegetables	10 minutes	1 hour

Each serving has:			
7 g carbohydrate	2 g fiber		32 g protein

¼ cup olive oil

8 pork chops, about ½ in. thick

2 medium onions, sliced

1 clove garlic, chopped

1 (28-oz.) can tomatoes (2½ to 3 cups)

1 head cabbage (about 2 lb.), coarsely shredded

1 tsp. salt

⅛ tsp. pepper

⅛ tsp. dried sage

1 cup dry red wine

1. Preheat the oven to 350°F.

2. Heat oil over medium heat in a large skillet. Brown chops 3 minutes on each side. Remove to an oven-proof casserole dish.

3. In the same skillet, sauté onions and garlic 3 minutes. Stir in tomatoes, and add cabbage, salt, pepper, sage, and wine. Spread mixture over chops.

4. Bake for 60 minutes or until cabbage and chops are tender. Check occasionally. You can prepare this in advance and refrigerate up to 2 days.

RECIPE FOR SUCCESS

The chops turn out tender and delicious with the taste of cabbage in the red wine. This recipe has two servings of vegetables, so consider this dish a complete meal.

Marinated Pork Tenderloin

Yield:	Serving size:	Prep time:	Cook time:
10 servings	4 ounces	15 minutes plus 24 hours marinating time	2½ hours

Each serving has:			
1 g carbohydrate	< 1 g fiber	30 g protein	

½ cup dry white wine	2 TB. butter
¼ cup olive oil	½ tsp. celery seed
6 TB. Dijon mustard	½ tsp. salt
¼ cup white mushrooms, chopped	½ tsp. freshly ground black pepper
2 TB. soy sauce	1 (5-lb.) pork loin roast, boned, rolled, and tied
2 TB. fresh lemon juice	
2 TB. onion, minced	

1. In a large bowl, mix together wine, oil, mustard, mushrooms, soy sauce, lemon juice, onion, butter, celery seed, salt, and pepper. Place pork roast in a rectangular baking pan, and pour marinade over meat. Cover and refrigerate 24 hours, turning occasionally.

2. Preheat oven to 350°F.

3. Place tenderloin with marinade into a roasting pan. Roast at 350°F for 2½ hours or to an internal temperature of 155°F to 160°F.

RECIPE FOR SUCCESS

If you haven't cooked with pork tenderloin before, now is the time. The meat is tender, lean, and loves to take up the flavors of spices and mushrooms. You'll soon become friends with this tasty cut of pork.

Pork Chops with Spaghetti

Yield:	Serving size:	Prep time:	Cook time:
4 servings	1 (6-ounce) pork chop with $\frac{1}{2}$ cup squash	20 minutes	1 hour

Each serving has:		
12 g carbohydrate	3 g fiber	21 g protein

1 spaghetti squash	$\frac{1}{8}$ tsp. crushed red pepper
4 ($\frac{3}{4}$-in. thick) pork chops	1 tsp. dried rosemary
$\frac{1}{2}$ cup butter (1 stick)	2 cups tomatoes, chopped
4 TB. Parmesan cheese, grated	$\frac{1}{4}$ cup fresh parsley, chopped
$\frac{1}{2}$ tsp. garlic, minced	$\frac{1}{2}$ tsp. salt
$\frac{1}{4}$ tsp. freshly ground black pepper	

1. Preheat the oven to 350°F.

2. Place spaghetti squash in a baking dish, and bake for 1 to $1\frac{1}{2}$ hours or until done. To test for doneness, prick skin with a fork. If the fork enters easily, squash is done. While squash is baking, prepare pork chops.

3. Melt 4 tablespoons butter in a large, heavy skillet. Add garlic, black pepper, red pepper, and rosemary. Add pork chops and brown slowly. Add tomatoes, parsley, and salt. Cover and simmer for 20 minutes. Uncover and cook 20 more minutes until pork chops are tender.

4. When squash is tender when pricked with a fork, split open with a knife and scoop out and discard seeds. Take a fork and scrape inside of squash. The flesh comes out in strands—like spaghetti. Toss strands with 4 tablespoons butter and Parmesan cheese.

5. Place spaghetti squash strands on a platter, arrange chops on spaghetti, and pour sauce over all.

TABLE TALK

You can also cook the spaghetti squash in the microwave as you would a baked potato. Prick the skin with a fork in several places. Microwave on high for 12 to 15 minutes. Cut open and scoop out seeds. Then use a fork to separate and remove the strands from the shells.

Pork Chops with Raisins and Walnuts

Yield:	Serving size:	Prep time:	Cook time:
4 servings	1 pork chop	10 minutes plus 2 to 3 hours marinating time	20 minutes

Each serving has:		
5 g carbohydrate	1 g fiber	20 g protein

4 (¾-in. thick) pork chops

¼ cup bourbon

½ cup water

2 TB. apple juice

¼ tsp. cayenne

¼ tsp. freshly ground black pepper

1 clove garlic, minced

2 TB. raisins

¼ cup walnuts

1. Place pork chops, bourbon, water, apple juice, cayenne, pepper, garlic, raisins, and walnuts into a large, resealable plastic bag. Marinate 2 to 3 hours at room temperature or overnight in the refrigerator.

2. When you are ready to cook, move pork chops to a heavy skillet and fry until cooked through. At the same time, put marinade—including raisins and walnuts (they're the best part!)—into a small saucepan. Bring to a boil and reduce sauce to ½ volume.

3. Remove pork chops to a serving platter and pour sauce over pork chops.

 RECIPE FOR SUCCESS

This recipe has a surprising flavor. The bourbon imparts a great and unusual taste, but don't worry about the alcohol—it evaporates during cooking. And the walnuts taste so good!

Veal Chops with Tarragon

Yield:	Serving size:	Prep time:	Cook time:
4 servings	1 veal chop	20 minutes	10 minutes

Each serving has:		
2 g carbohydrate	0 g fiber	20 g protein

4 veal chops, about ¾- to 1-in. thick

4 TB. olive oil

2 TB. lemon juice

2 tsp. dried tarragon

¼ cup butter (½ stick)

1 TB. fresh tarragon, chopped, or 1 tsp. dried tarragon

¼ tsp. garlic, minced

¼ tsp. salt

¼ tsp. pepper

1. Place veal chops in a resealable plastic bag. Put in olive oil, lemon juice, and 1 teaspoon tarragon. Close the bag and marinate 2 to 3 hours or overnight in the refrigerator. Turn over the bag occasionally to marinate chops on all sides.

2. To make tarragon butter, melt butter in the microwave with 1 teaspoon tarragon, garlic, salt, and pepper. Set aside.

3. Heat a heavy skillet and brown chops. Cook for about 4 minutes per side, basting with marinade. Serve topped with tarragon butter.

Variation: Substitute basil for tarragon in this recipe. It will be just as delicious.

RECIPE FOR SUCCESS

These veal chops are easy to prepare. They are quite tender when marinated and cooked or grilled quickly. Serve for special occasions and to special guests.

Curried Pork Chops with Apricots

Yield:	Serving size:	Prep time:	Cook time:
4 servings	1 pork chop	30 minutes with ¼ cup sauce	40 minutes

Each serving has:		
6 g carbohydrate	< 1 g fiber	19 g protein

1 medium onion, chopped	4 pork chops
3 TB. butter	4 dried apricot halves, chopped
1 TB. flour	¼ cup water
1 TB. curry powder	1 cup sliced white mushrooms
¾ cup white wine	6 TB. butter
Salt and pepper to taste	

1. Make sauce first. Sauté onions in butter until just tender. Sprinkle with flour, and add curry powder. Cook 1 to 2 minutes, stirring, and add white wine. Season with salt and pepper. Simmer while cooking pork chops.

2. Put chopped apricots and water into a small bowl, and microwave for 1 minute, until water boils. Remove and let stand to let apricots get tender and soft.

3. Sauté mushrooms over high heat in 3 tablespoons butter. In a separate skillet, sauté pork chops in remaining 3 tablespoons butter until browned on both sides.

4. Top pork chops with apricots, then curry sauce. Season with salt and pepper. Spread mushrooms over sauce, cover the skillet, and cook gently for 30 minutes or until done.

RECIPE FOR SUCCESS

The apricots and mushrooms enhance the mild curry taste. But don't let it fool you; the combination makes your mouth sing. And it sure doesn't taste like low carb.

Pork Chops with Apples

Yield:	Serving size:	Prep time:	Cook time:
4 servings	1 pork chop and 1 apple	20 minutes	10 to 15 minutes

Each serving has:		
15 g carbohydrate	5 g fiber	19 g protein

4 (¾-in. thick) pork chops

3 TB. butter

3 medium cooking apples, such as Fuji, Golden Delicious, or Granny Smith

Salt and pepper to taste

1. Preheat the oven to 300°F.

2. Sauté pork chops on both sides in butter to brown and then continue cooking at a high temperature for 10 minutes, turning once after 5 minutes.

3. Core apples and cut into thin slices. Leave skins on.

4. Arrange pork chops in a shallow oven dish, and pour pan juices over chops. Arrange apple slices around chops. Season with salt and pepper. Bake for about 10 to 15 minutes, until apples are tender.

RECIPE FOR SUCCESS

With just 3 ingredients plus salt and pepper, you can make these interesting pork chops. They are sweet with a light tang from the apples.

Pork Chops with Sauerkraut

Yield:	Serving size:	Prep time:	Cook time:
6 servings	1 pork chop and $\frac{1}{2}$ cup sauerkraut	15 minutes	1 hour

Each serving has:		
5 g carbohydrate	4 g fiber	20 g protein

6 pork chops, $\frac{3}{4}$- to 1-in. thick

3 TB. butter

2 lb. sauerkraut, drained

1 TB. molasses

$\frac{1}{4}$ cup water

$\frac{1}{4}$ tsp. caraway seeds

$\frac{1}{4}$ tsp. freshly ground black pepper

1. Preheat the oven to 350°F.

2. Sauté pork chops in butter to brown on both sides.

3. Mix sauerkraut, molasses, water, caraway seeds, and pepper in an oven casserole. Place pork chops on top of mixture. Cover and bake about 1 hour.

RECIPE FOR SUCCESS

Sauerkraut, notably low in carbs, gives the pork chops a highly tangy and interesting flavor. The caraway seeds add authenticity to this recipe, adapted from Middle European cuisine. Baked apples are a great accompaniment.

Oven BBQ Ribs

Yield:	Serving size:	Prep time:	Cook time:
6 servings	Approximately 5 to 6 ribs	15 minutes	1 hour 15 minutes

Each serving has:		
12 g carbohydrate	0 g fiber	21 g protein

6 lb. spareribs, cut into serving-size pieces

Boiling water

1 cup ketchup

⅓ cup Worcestershire sauce

2 TB. soy sauce

½ cup water

¼ cup lemon juice

4 to 5 dashes hot pepper sauce

2 onions, minced

2 cloves garlic, minced

1 tsp. paprika

1 tsp. dry mustard

1 tsp. black pepper

¼ tsp. ginger

1. Preheat the oven to 450°F.

2. *Parboil* ribs in a large pot for 5 minutes. Drain and set aside.

3. Combine ketchup, Worcestershire sauce, soy sauce, water, lemon juice, hot pepper sauce, onions, garlic, paprika, mustard, black pepper, and ginger in a saucepan. Bring to a boil, reduce heat, and simmer until thickened.

4. While sauce simmers, line a roasting pan with heavy foil, and place ribs on the foil and cover. Bake for 15 minutes, and remove from the oven. Reduce heat to 350°F. Pour sauce over ribs, covering well. Cover the pan with foil, and bake 1 hour. Check every 15 minutes, basting as needed.

DEFINITION

Parboil means to boil partially or for a short time. In this recipe, parboiling the ribs removes some of the fat and precooks them.

Green Tomatoes and Ham

Yield:	Serving size:	Prep time:	Cook time:
6 servings	4 ounces ham with ½ cup vegetables	15 minutes	40 minutes

Each serving has:		
11 g carbohydrate	2 g fiber	27 g protein

1 (2-lb.) (or 2 smaller) ham slice, ¾ in. thick, fully cooked

5 medium green tomatoes, sliced ¼ in. thick

3 onions, sliced ¼ in. thick

2 TB. Worcestershire sauce

2 TB. brown sugar

1 tsp. tarragon

1 tsp. dry mustard

½ tsp. black pepper

1. Preheat the oven to 350°F.

2. On top of the stove, brown ham on both sides; place in the bottom of a baking dish. Place tomato and onion slices on top of ham; sprinkle with Worcestershire sauce, brown sugar, tarragon, mustard, and black pepper. Cover dish and bake 40 minutes.

RECIPE FOR SUCCESS

This is a deliciously simple dish ready to eat in under an hour. Use your favorite seasonings to make this dish uniquely yours. Top the ham with bell pepper rings to give additional flavor, or try sprinkling with a bit of cinnamon or basil.

Mushroom-Gingered Ham Slice

Yield:	Serving size:	Prep time:	Cook time:
6 servings	5 ounces with ¼ cup sauce	20 minutes plus 1 hour marinating time ham	40 minutes

Each serving has:		
7 g carbohydrate	2 g fiber	25 g protein

1 tsp. dry mustard	2 cloves garlic, minced
1 tsp. ground ginger	1 stalk celery, sliced
½ cup white wine	1 cup heavy cream
2 lb. ham slice, 1 to 2 in. thick, fully cooked	1 (8-oz.) can button mushrooms or 1 pint fresh mushrooms, sliced
5 TB. butter	1 TB. cornstarch
1 large onion, minced	¼ cup water

1. Preheat the oven to 425°F.

2. Blend together mustard, ginger, and wine, and pour over ham slice. Refrigerate for 1 hour, turning occasionally.

3. Drain ham, reserving liquid. Melt 2 tablespoons butter in a skillet and brown ham. Remove ham, place in a baking dish, and set aside. In the same skillet, melt remaining 3 tablespoons butter, if needed, to sauté onions, garlic, and celery.

4. When vegetables are tender, add marinade and cream to the skillet; heat to simmering, stir in mushrooms, and simmer 10 minutes.

5. Mix cornstarch into water to form smooth paste, and slowly stir into sauce mixture, cooking and stirring constantly until thickened. Pour over ham slice in the baking dish, and bake 20 minutes.

RECIPE FOR SUCCESS

This ham dish offers a delectable and unusual taste treat. Serve with salad and a vegetable, such as asparagus, green beans, or peas.

Smothered Pork Chops

Yield:	Serving size:	Prep time:	Cook time:
6 servings	1 pork chop	15 minutes	1 hour

Each serving has:		
5 g carbohydrate	2 g fiber	21 g protein

1 TB. butter	2 cups chicken broth
6 pork chops, 1 in. thick	1 cup sliced carrots
2 large onions, chopped	1 TB. cornstarch
½ bell pepper, chopped	¼ cup water
1 tsp. garlic, minced	1 tsp. Worcestershire sauce

1. Melt butter in a skillet, and brown pork chops on both sides. Remove from the pan and set aside. In the same skillet, sauté onions, bell pepper, and garlic until tender. Add chicken broth and carrots to the skillet, and bring to a simmer.

2. Mix cornstarch into water, and stir to a smooth paste; add to the skillet, and stir to thicken. Add Worcestershire sauce and pork chops to the skillet. Cover and cook over low heat for 1 hour or until meat is cooked.

Veal Parmesan

Yield:	Serving size:	Prep time:	Cook time:
6 servings	4 ounces	20 minutes	30 minutes

Each serving has:		
10 g carbohydrate	3 g fiber	30 g protein

3 TB. butter	¼ tsp. Italian herb mixture
1 onion, minced	1 lb. veal cutlets, thinly sliced
3 cloves garlic, minced	¾ cup Parmesan cheese
1 (28-oz.) can Italian-seasoned tomato pieces	¼ cup breadcrumbs, finely ground
1 (8-oz.) can tomato sauce	1 large egg, slightly beaten
Salt and pepper to taste	3 TB. olive oil
¼ tsp. dried basil	½ lb. mozzarella cheese slices

1. Preheat the oven to 350°F.

2. Melt butter in a skillet and sauté onion and garlic until tender. Add tomatoes, tomato sauce, salt, pepper, basil, and herb mixture; simmer 10 minutes.

3. Pound cutlets until very thin. Combine ½ cup Parmesan cheese and breadcrumbs. Dip cutlets into egg and then into breading mixture, covering well. In a separate skillet, heat olive oil and brown cutlets on both sides.

4. In one layer, place cutlets in a large baking dish, and pour ⅔ sauce over top. Layer mozzarella slices over sauce, and pour remaining tomato sauce on top of cheese. Sprinkle remaining Parmesan cheese over all and bake, uncovered, for 30 minutes.

TABLE TALK

This recipe is a classic Italian favorite that's also low carb. Serve with spaghetti squash and sliced tomatoes on lettuce. It's wonderful because you get the terrific tastes of the Mediterranean without the pasta.

RECIPE FOR SUCCESS

This hearty pork dish includes plenty of vegetables. Add a tossed salad with a mild dressing such as Ranch or poppyseed to balance the savory taste of the sauce.

The Least You Need to Know

- Pork is a delicious meat that can be prepared in a wide variety of intriguing ways.
- Pork cuts can be low fat or high fat. Let your taste preferences guide you.
- Veal and pork are light meats that take well to marinating or tenderizing with other recipe ingredients.
- Cook pork to a minimum internal temperature of 137°F, and clean work areas thoroughly.
- Pork and veal contain no carbohydrates and offer complete protein, so they are great for low-carb eating.

Chapter 10

Poultry Main Dishes

In This Chapter

- The ease of cooking with chicken
- Interchanging chicken and turkey
- Tasty and varied low-carb meals with chicken

Perhaps you most enjoy the breast meat of a chicken or turkey. Or maybe you love the dark meat and delight in savoring the turkey legs at Thanksgiving. Whichever part you prefer, recipes in this chapter can satisfy your appetite.

Chicken is the most adaptable of meats. It can be roasted, stewed, sautéed, or cooked on the grill. And it can even be baked on top of an opened can of beer!

Chicken has a comparatively mild, almost bland taste, so it readily takes on the flavors of other ingredients in a recipe. Here you'll find recipes for chicken combined with a wide variety of both sweet and hot spices, plus many different fruits, meats, and condiments. Chicken contains less fat than other meats so you can cook it with butter and cream to create a richer taste or with water or bouillon for a lighter-tasting meal.

Another No-Carb Food

Chicken has no carbohydrates. Hooray! Rather, it contains high-quality complete protein and both saturated and unsaturated fats. So chicken cooked without other ingredients is totally carb free. Unfortunately, eating plain chicken without other ingredients would get boring really fast. It would also eliminate lots of wonderful, delicious chicken meals.

It's the other ingredients in these recipes that add to the carb count. These ingredients include fruits, spices, condiments, nuts, and vegetables plus some flour or cornstarch used as thickeners. We have minimized the use of thickeners, and you can omit them if you want to reduce the carb count further. But as you can tell by glancing through these recipes, the carb count is already low and should meet your requirements for low-carb meals.

TABLE TALK

We figure that if you're going to spend your time cooking a delicious chicken meal, you may as well make plenty so you can have leftovers for breakfast or lunch the next day. Best of all, you can relax about what low-carb meal to have the next day for breakfast and/or lunch. Because many of the recipes taste great cold as well as heated, they are perfect for sack lunches.

What Goes with Chicken (or Turkey)

As you plan your chicken meals, always make sure you have two servings of either fruits and/or vegetables at your meal. For instance, serve a tossed salad and steamed vegetable for a wholesome, delicious, and balanced meal. Or substitute fresh fruit for the salad.

You want to "eat a rainbow" as best you can at every meal, so think of side dishes with tomatoes, green vegetables, colorful salad greens, in-season fruit, or a tangy salsa.

And if you have room left in your stomach, add in a treat from the dessert or chocolate recipes in Chapters 24 and 25, respectively.

With the exception of Roast Turkey, we have written all the recipes in this chapter using chicken, but you can substitute turkey for all these recipes except Beer Bottom Smoked Chicken. We don't want you to impale a turkey on that can of beer. Use a chicken only for that recipe, please.

Otherwise, choose turkey or chicken based on what sounds good to you that day. Turkey is a tasty alternative that adds variety and can be quite economical.

Paprika Chicken

Yield:	Serving size:	Prep time:	Cook time:
6 servings	½ breast	30 minutes	40 minutes

Each serving has:		
5 g carbohydrate	1 g fiber	29 g protein

3 TB. butter	5 strips bacon, cooked and coarsely crumbled
3 chicken breasts (1 lb.), boned, skinned, and halved	1 cup dry white wine
2 large onions, chopped coarsely	2 cups water
1 clove garlic, minced	½ tsp. salt
2 cups white mushrooms, cut in quarters	¼ tsp. pepper
	Pinch cayenne
2 TB. paprika	¾ cup heavy cream

1. Heat butter in a heavy pan and sauté chicken, onions, garlic, and mushrooms until chicken is well browned on all sides. Sprinkle with paprika. Add bacon, white wine, and enough water to cover. Season with salt, pepper, and a small pinch of cayenne. Cover the pan and cook about 35 minutes.

2. Remove chicken pieces with a slotted spoon and boil sauce down until slightly thick. Put chicken back into sauce. Add cream, stir, and taste for seasoning.

RECIPE FOR SUCCESS

Family and friends will exclaim, "This is chicken?!" This decadently rich dish with its creamy sauce has a deep reddish-brown color. When we serve this at a party, friends seem to end up licking the serving bowl. You can substitute water for the wine, if you like. This is a rich and hearty main dish, so serve with lighter fare, such as a fresh salad with a tangy dressing and a side of steamed veggies with butter.

Pine Nut Chicken

Yield:	Serving size:	Prep time:	Cook time:
8 servings	1 breast	20 minutes	35 minutes
Each serving has:			
6 g carbohydrate	1 g fiber	38 g protein	

1½ cups pine nuts, finely chopped

3 TB. cornmeal

2 TB. fresh basil, chopped

2 cloves garlic, minced

½ tsp. dried sage

½ tsp. cayenne

¼ tsp. salt

1 large egg white

3 TB. Dijon mustard

1½ tsp. water

8 boneless, skinless chicken breast halves, or thighs

1. Preheat the oven to 375°F, and grease a large baking dish.

2. Combine pine nuts, cornmeal, basil, garlic, sage, cayenne, and salt in a bowl. Add egg white and stir. Transfer to a shallow dish.

3. In a small bowl, combine mustard and water. Spread mixture evenly over chicken. Roll chicken in pine nut mixture, and press to coat evenly. Arrange in the baking dish.

4. Bake until coating is crisp and browned, about 35 minutes.

TABLE TALK

Pine nuts come from the piñon pine tree, which grows wild in the southwestern United States and in Mediterranean countries. They contain more protein per weight than any other nut.

RECIPE FOR SUCCESS

If you are not familiar with pine nuts, then you need to get familiar! They have a delightful taste. That said, you can use other nuts in place of the pine nuts. Select from pecans, almonds, walnuts, or peanuts, and the carb count stays basically the same. Make ahead and serve cold for picnics and outings. Try this recipe with Fiesta Confetti Salsa (see recipe in Chapter 20) and a side dish of spicy green beans.

Chicken Stir-Fry with Fruit

Yield:	Serving size:	Prep time:	Cook time:
6 servings	¾ cup	20 minutes plus marinate for 2 hours	10 minutes

Each serving has:		
6 g carbohydrate	2 g fiber	23 g protein

2 tsp. white wine

1 tsp. soy sauce

¼ tsp. fresh ginger, peeled and grated

1 tsp. cornstarch

½ tsp. salt

¼ tsp. pepper

3 boneless, skinless chicken breasts, cut into strips

½ cup snow peas

4 green onions, sliced

3 TB. peanut oil

1 cup green grapes

1 cup cantaloupe, cubed

1 TB. garlic, minced

⅓ cup peanuts, chopped

1. Combine white wine, soy sauce, ginger, cornstarch, salt, and pepper in a bowl and mix well. Add chicken to this mixture, and refrigerate for 2 hours or longer.

2. Slice snow peas and onions diagonally into ½-inch pieces.

3. Heat a wok or a large skillet over high heat for 45 seconds. Add 1 tablespoon peanut oil, and swirl evenly to coat. Add snow peas and onions. Stir-fry for 1 minute or until snow peas are bright green. Add grapes and cantaloupe. Stir-fry for 1 minute. Remove with a slotted spoon, and wipe the wok with a paper towel.

4. Reheat the wok, add 2 tablespoons peanut oil, and heat. Add garlic and stir-fry for 30 seconds. Add chicken and cook 2 minutes or more, stirring until cooked through.

5. Return fruit and vegetables to the wok. Cook for 1 minute until heated through. Serve immediately. Garnish with peanuts.

RECIPE FOR SUCCESS

Cantaloupe isn't just for breakfast! Melon can be cooked quickly, as in stir-frying. You can substitute other fruits, such as pineapple, raisins, apples, and papaya for the fruit in this recipe. Other nuts such as walnuts, cashews, pecans, pine nuts, almonds, or even macadamias will work as substitutes for the peanuts. This is a meal all by itself, but if you want more, go with a low-carb side dish like a salad or a simple vegetable like sliced tomatoes.

Rosemary Roasted Chicken

Yield:	Serving size:	Prep time:	Cook time:
6 servings	1 breast or 1 leg and thigh	10 minutes	60 minutes

Each serving has:			
8 g carbohydrate	0 g fiber	25 g protein	

4-lb. baking chicken

Salt and freshly ground pepper to taste

3 cloves garlic, cut into halves

4 sprigs fresh rosemary

1 TB. fresh rosemary, chopped or 1 to 2 tsp. dried

1. Preheat the oven to 400°F.

2. Remove giblets and neck from chicken cavity. Rinse chicken and pat dry. Season inside and out with a generous mixture of salt and pepper. Put garlic and rosemary sprigs in the cavity, and pat chopped rosemary on the outside of chicken.

3. Place chicken, breast side down, on a rack in a roasting pan. Bake for 30 minutes, basting with pan juices every 10 minutes. Turn chicken breast side up, and roast for 30 minutes longer or until chicken is cooked through and the outside is crisp and brown.

RECIPE FOR SUCCESS

Don't be timid with rosemary! Rosemary is a wonderfully aromatic herb, and the kitchen will be filled with a wonderful fragrance as the chicken bakes. The recipe is also terrific if you substitute tarragon for the rosemary. This dish is perfect for dinner or a picnic. For a great side dish, serve asparagus with hollandaise sauce.

Chicken with Olives and Capers

Yield:	Serving size:	Prep time:	Cook time:
8 servings	1 breast or 1 leg and thigh	20 minutes plus marinate overnight	1 hour

Each serving has:		
5 g carbohydrate	< 1 g fiber	32 g protein

2 (2½-lb.) chickens, cut into pieces

1 TB. garlic, minced

2 TB. dried oregano

1 tsp. salt

½ tsp. freshly ground pepper to taste

¼ cup red wine vinegar

¼ cup olive oil

½ cup dried apricot halves

¼ cup pitted green olives

¼ cup capers

3 bay leaves

½ cup white wine

¼ cup fresh parsley, chopped

1. In a large bowl, combine chicken, garlic, oregano, salt, pepper, vinegar, olive oil, apricots, olives, capers, and bay leaves. Cover and let marinate, refrigerated overnight.

2. The next day, preheat the oven to 350°F.

3. Arrange chicken in a single layer in 1 or 2 shallow baking pans, and spoon marinade evenly over chicken. Pour white wine into pan(s).

4. Bake for 1 hour, basting frequently with pan juices. Chicken is done when thigh pieces, pricked with a fork, have a clear yellow rather than a pink juice.

5. To serve, remove bay leaf and sprinkle chicken with parsley. Serve pan juices separately.

RECIPE FOR SUCCESS

Expect to hear a few "Wows!" with this recipe. It's great for a buffet dinner because the chicken is so tender your guests can easily cut it with a spoon (just in case you run out of knives and forks!). The recipe can be doubled or tripled for a crowd. You can substitute a little water for the white wine. Because this is a rich and hearty main course, select light and rather plain side dishes, such as a tossed salad and steamed vegetables.

Italian Baked Chicken

Yield:	Serving size:	Prep time:	Cook time:
6 servings	½ breast	15 minutes	25 minutes
Each serving has:			
< 1 g carbohydrate	0 g fiber	21 g protein	

½ cup Parmesan cheese, freshly grated

2 TB. fresh parsley, minced

½ tsp. garlic, minced

1 tsp. dried oregano

1 tsp. dried basil

¼ tsp. crushed red pepper

½ tsp. freshly ground black pepper

3 chicken breasts, boned, skinned, and halved

3 TB. butter, melted

1. Preheat the oven to 375°F.

2. Combine Parmesan, parsley, garlic, oregano, basil, red pepper, and black pepper in a shallow dish. Dip chicken into melted butter and then into cheese mixture. Place into a shallow baking pan. Drizzle remaining butter over chicken, and sprinkle with any remaining cheese mixture.

3. Bake for 25 minutes or until tender.

RECIPE FOR SUCCESS

Delicious served hot or cold, this dish can be on the table in less than an hour. The Parmesan cheese and spices add some low-carb zing to the chicken. Serve with a Caesar salad and steamed vegetables such as broccoli, brussels sprouts, or green beans.

Chicken Piccata

Yield:	Serving size:	Prep time:	Cook time:
6 servings	½ breast	10 minutes	15 minutes

Each serving has:			
4 g carbohydrate	< 1 g fiber	22 g protein	

3 whole chicken breasts, boned, skinned, and halved

3 TB. flour

¼ tsp. salt

¼ tsp. pepper

¼ cup butter

½ cup white wine

¼ cup fresh-squeezed lemon juice

2 TB. capers

1. Pound chicken between 2 sheets of waxed paper until ¼ inch thick. Dredge chicken in flour that has been seasoned with salt and pepper.

2. Melt butter in a heavy skillet until sizzling. Sauté chicken breasts in butter until light brown, about 3 minutes per side. Add wine, lemon juice, and capers to chicken, and let boil 3 minutes or until cooked thoroughly, turning chicken in sauce.

3. Arrange chicken on a platter. Serve with sauce drizzled on top.

Variation: Veal Piccata is another wonderful way to get the piccata flavor into your mouth. Substitute veal in this recipe, and the amount of carbohydrates stays the same.

TABLE TALK

Eating foods that are acidic lowers the glycemic index of the food. The lower the glycemic index, the less it increases blood sugar levels in the body, which is what you want to avoid by eating low carb. This recipe contains capers, which are acidic.

RECIPE FOR SUCCESS

The tanginess of the lemon juice and capers creates the magical taste of this dish. Serve garnished with lemon wedges and fresh parsley. Recommended side dishes are spaghetti squash with tomato sauce and tossed salad with Italian vinaigrette. Or complete your meal with steamed carrots with zucchini and red peppers sprinkled with oregano or basil.

Curried Chicken

Yield:	Serving size:	Prep time:	Cook time:
6 servings	1 breast or 1 leg and thigh	10 minutes	20 minutes

Each serving has:			
7 g carbohydrate	1 g fiber	29 g protein	

1 large onion, chopped coarsely

3 TB. butter

1 (3-lb.) chicken, cut into pieces

2 cups chicken bouillon

$\frac{1}{2}$ tsp. garlic, minced

1 tsp. salt

$\frac{1}{2}$ tsp. freshly ground pepper

1 TB. curry powder

1 green pepper, cut into $\frac{1}{2}$-in. squares

$\frac{1}{2}$ cup sliced fresh peaches

2 TB. raisins

3 TB. almonds, slivered

1. In a large skillet, sauté onion in 2 tablespoons butter. Add chicken and brown. Add chicken bouillon, and stir until slightly thickened. Add garlic, salt, pepper, and curry powder; cook over medium-low heat for 15 to 20 minutes.

2. In a separate skillet, sauté green pepper, peaches, and raisins in remaining 1 tablespoon butter until warmed and soft. Serve chicken with fruit sauce, and sprinkle with slivered almonds.

RECIPE FOR SUCCESS

To lower the carb count, you can omit the fruit sauce but keep the slivered almonds. You can also serve the following condiments with the curried chicken without increasing the carb count much: chopped hard-cooked eggs, shredded coconut, chopped black or green olives, chopped salted peanuts, chopped crisp bacon. If you add the following condiments, the carb count does increase: orange marmalade, store-bought chutney, sweet pickle relish, crushed pineapple.

Artichoke Chicken with Mushrooms

Yield:	Serving size:	Prep time:	Cook time:
6 servings	1 breast or 1 leg and thigh	15 minutes	1 hour

Each serving has:			
7 g carbohydrate with sherry or 3 g carbohydrate with broth	2 g fiber	34 g protein	

1 (2- to 3-lb.) chicken, cut into pieces
Salt and pepper to taste
2 TB. butter
½ lb. crimini mushrooms, sliced
½ cup sherry or chicken broth

2 TB. lemon or lime juice
1 (14-oz.) can artichokes, drained
1 cup heavy cream
½ cup sliced green onions
½ cup plain yogurt, such as Greek yogurt

1. Season chicken pieces with salt and pepper. Melt butter in a large skillet. Brown chicken on both sides, about 5 minutes per side. Add mushrooms, sherry, and lemon juice.

2. Bring to a boil, and reduce heat to a simmer. Cover and cook 45 minutes or until chicken is done. Add artichokes and cream and stir, cooking for 5 more minutes. Mix in green onions and yogurt. Let simmer until hot.

RECIPE FOR SUCCESS

We love the combination of artichokes, mushrooms, and chicken—they seem made for each other. To make this recipe lower in fat (but higher in carbs), you can substitute evaporated skim milk for the heavy cream and use low-fat yogurt instead of plain yogurt.

Basil Stuffed Chicken

Yield:	Serving size:	Prep time:	Cook time:
6 servings	¼ chicken	25 minutes	60 minutes

Each serving has:		
3 g carbohydrate	0 g fiber	35 g protein

2 TB. butter

½ onion, chopped

4 cloves garlic, chopped

3 TB. fresh basil leaves or 1 TB. dried basil

1 large egg

½ cup Swiss cheese, shredded

Black pepper to taste

6 chicken quarters, leave skin intact

1. Preheat the oven to 400°F.

2. Melt butter in a 2-quart pan over medium heat. Sauté onion and garlic, and cook until tender, about 2 minutes, stirring often. Remove from heat; add basil, egg, cheese, and pepper.

3. Carefully loosen chicken skin on each quarter by pushing your finger between skin and meat to form a pocket. Spoon stuffing into each pocket.

4. Place chicken in a 9 × 13-inch buttered baking dish, and bake 50 minutes or until tender.

RECIPE FOR SUCCESS

You can use spinach, curly parsley, cilantro, or shredded zucchini in place of the basil. Put a baked yellow squash casserole in the oven to cook with the chicken and your meal is complete.

Beer Bottom Smoked Chicken

Yield:	Serving size:	Prep time:	Cook time:
6 servings	1 breast or 1 leg and thigh	20 minutes, plus 6 hours marinating time	2 hours

Each serving has:		
2 g carbohydrate	0 g fiber	32 g protein

½ cup lime juice

½ cup orange juice

⅓ cup olive oil

1 TB. garlic, minced

¼ cup fresh cilantro, minced

½ tsp. cayenne

1 jalapeño pepper, minced and
seeded (or amount desired)

Salt and pepper to taste

1 (2- to 3-lb.) whole chicken

1 can light beer

1. Mix together lime juice, orange juice, olive oil, garlic, cilantro, cayenne, jalapeño, salt, and pepper. Use amount of jalapeños as desired for your taste. Remove and refrigerate ½ cup marinade to use for basting during grilling.

2. Wash chicken and remove and throw away gizzards, etc. Place chicken in a large resealable plastic bag, and pour in marinade. Squeeze excess air from the bag, and refrigerate at least 6 hours or overnight. Turn occasionally. Discard marinade when removing chicken for cooking.

3. Preheat grill to medium-hot. Place a roasting pan on the grill. Open beer can, and carefully insert can into chicken cavity. Push chicken onto can so it will not tip over on the grill. Set can and chicken in the roasting pan on the grill off the direct fire, and close the grill cover.

4. Beer will boil during cooking, basting chicken on the inside.

5. Grill chicken about 2 hours or until a meat thermometer inserted into the thickest portion of chicken registers 180°F.

 RECIPE FOR SUCCESS

This is a terrific recipe for party cooking—it makes for quite a lively and, perhaps, silly discussion. The double basting causes the chicken to be very moist.

Chinese Chicken

Yield:	Serving size:	Prep time:	Cook time:
6 servings	1 cup	35 minutes, plus cooking time for chicken	20 minutes

Each serving has:			
9 g carbohydrate	1 g fiber	32 g protein	

3 cooked chicken breasts, shredded

2 TB. butter

1 cup celery, chopped

1 cup onion, chopped

2 cups chicken broth

1 TB. molasses

3 TB. soy sauce

1 (14-oz.) can Chinese vegetables, drained

1 (8-oz.) can bean sprouts, drained

Pepper to taste

1 (8-oz.) can sliced water chestnuts, drained

1 TB. cornstarch

1 cup water

1. Melt butter in a Dutch oven, and sauté celery and onion until tender. Add chicken broth, molasses, soy sauce, vegetables, bean sprouts, pepper, and water chestnuts to the pot. Simmer slowly until bubbly.

2. Add cornstarch to water, and stir until a paste forms. Slowly add paste to the pot, and stir to thicken to gravy consistency.

3. Add chicken and simmer 10 minutes.

RECIPE FOR SUCCESS

You may add additional vegetables to this recipe, such as fresh mushrooms, snow peas, or various colored bell peppers. You can substitute cooked beef for the chicken. Serve over a small serving of rice, if desired, which does increase carbohydrate count. Seasonal mixed fresh fruit is a delicious addition to a Chinese meal as well as a broth-based soup appetizer.

Chicken Macadamia

Yield:	Serving size:	Prep time:	Cook time:
6 servings	1 breast or 1 leg and thigh	15 minutes	45 minutes

Each serving has:			
4 g carbohydrate	2 g fiber	34 g protein	

2 large eggs, beaten	$\frac{1}{4}$ cup plus 1 cup cold water
2 TB. olive oil	2 to 3 chicken breasts, halved
2 TB. soy sauce	$\frac{1}{2}$ cup macadamia nuts, chopped
1 tsp. powdered ginger	$\frac{1}{2}$ medium green pepper, diced
$\frac{1}{4}$ tsp. pepper	$\frac{1}{2}$ medium red pepper, diced
2 TB. brandy	2 TB. cider vinegar
1 medium onion, minced	$\frac{1}{4}$ cup pineapple juice

1. Preheat the oven to 350°F.

2. Using a wire wisk, combine eggs, oil, soy sauce, ginger, pepper, brandy, onion, and $\frac{1}{4}$ cup water. Soak chicken in batter for at least 20 minutes. Dip in macadamia nut. Arrange chicken in an oven baking dish. Bake for 30-45 minutes until juices run clear.

3. While chicken is baking, make sauce. Place green and red peppers and 1 cup water in a saucepan, and bring to boil. Add vinegar and pineapple juice. Simmer.

4. Arrange warm chicken on a platter. Serve with sauce on the side.

RECIPE FOR SUCCESS

This recipe, with its Asian flavor, is so delicious that it's worth the effort. If preferred, use $\frac{1}{2}$ teaspoon brandy flavoring instead of the brandy.

Chicken Breasts Stuffed with Mushrooms and Spinach

Yield:	Serving size:	Prep time:	Cook time:
6 servings	1 breast	30 minutes	45 minutes
Each serving has:			
6 g carbohydrate	< 1 g fiber	38 g protein	

½ cup onion, chopped

½ tsp. crushed dried oregano

1 clove garlic, minced

6 TB. butter

4 cups fresh spinach

1 cup white mushrooms, chopped

4 TB. Parmesan cheese

4 oz. feta cheese

6 TB. red wine

6 boneless, skinless chicken breasts

6–12 toothpicks

1–2 TB. flour

⅓ cup heavy cream

¼ cup chicken broth

1 clove garlic, minced

2 TB. lemon juice

1 tsp. spicy mustard

Salt and pepper to taste

1. Preheat the oven to 350°F.

2. Sauté onion, oregano, and ½ minced garlic in 3 tablespoons butter. Add spinach and mushrooms; cook until spinach is wilted. Remove from heat.

3. Stir in Parmesan and feta cheeses and 3 tablespoons wine. Pound chicken breasts to flatten; divide stuffing and place in center of each breast. Wrap chicken around stuffing to form a roll. Secure with wooden toothpicks.

4. Lightly dust breasts with flour. Sauté in remaining 3 tablespoons butter until lightly browned; remove chicken to a baking dish, and bake for 30 minutes. Meanwhile, add cream, broth, remaining 3 tablespoons wine, remaining ½ minced garlic, lemon juice, mustard, salt, and pepper to pan juices; cook until sauce is slightly thickened.

5. Serve sauce over chicken.

RECIPE FOR SUCCESS

Steamed cauliflower makes a wonderful substitute for higher-carb potatoes. Steam cauliflower and mash, if desired, with a bit of butter and cream; serve with additional sauce as you would gravy and potatoes! Fresh strawberries make a colorful plate as well as give a touch of natural sweetness.

Roasted Turkey Breast

Yield:	Serving size:	Prep time:	Cook time:
6 servings	4 ounces	5 minutes	1 to 1½ hours
Each serving has:			
1 g carbohydrate	0 g fiber	25 g protein	

1 TB. dried rosemary	½ tsp. black pepper
1 tsp. garlic powder	1 (2-lb.) fresh turkey breast
1 tsp. dried thyme leaves	½ cup chicken broth or bouillon
1 tsp. dried oregano leaves	cube in water

1. Preheat the oven to 325°F.

2. Combine seasonings in a small dish.

3. Rinse turkey breast, dry, and place into a shallow baking dish on a rack or oven proof trivet. Add broth and water to just below upper rim of the baking dish.

4. Rub rosemary, garlic powder, thyme, oregano, and pepper onto turkey breast.

5. Bake 1 hour or until temperature registers 170°F on a meat thermometer.

 HOT POTATO

Cooking turkey until it registers 170°F on the thermometer is the safest way to be sure it is well done. Poultry is not a meat we eat medium-rare! A good rule of thumb is to cook about 20 minutes per pound.

The Least You Need to Know

- Chicken and turkey contain no carbohydrates and plenty of complete protein.
- Chicken and turkey are complemented by a wide variety of flavors, from tangy and spicy to sweet and fruity.
- For side dishes, add two or more vegetables and/or fruits.
- Leftover chicken dishes make for yummy breakfasts and lunches.
- You can substitute turkey for chicken in all the recipes in this chapter except Beer Bottom Smoked Chicken.

Seafood Main Dishes

In This Chapter

- Making seafood a part of your low-carb eating
- Cooking seafood with many different flavors
- Enjoying the rich taste of seafood

Seafood is our no-carb treat from the oceans. The many varieties of seafood—shrimp, crab, crawfish, and lobster just to name a few—can make eating low carb an absolute delight and are certainly anything but boring.

Cooked plain and served with drawn butter and some fresh lemon wedges, seafood is wonderful. It adds flavor when included in a recipe with, among others, sun-dried tomatoes, artichokes, or fennel.

Low-carb seafood recipes are great to make if you thrive on a busy lifestyle. They are easy to prepare and quick to make because seafood cooks in just minutes.

Ingredients for Seafood

Seafood tastes best with the best ingredients. These recipes call for the following kinds of ingredients:

- **Heavy cream.** Many of the recipes call for cream. Be sure to use real cream and do not substitute fake cream, milk, skim milk, or even half-and-half. The results will be puny, and quite frankly, you will have wasted your money on purchasing the seafood.

- **Sun-dried tomatoes.** You can purchase sun-dried tomatoes in oil by the jar and also dried in plastic or cellophane bags. For these recipes, it's easiest to use sun-dried tomatoes straight from the jar, but you can reconstitute the ones in bags by soaking them in warm water until they plump.

- **Butter.** Always use real butter. Only butter will do, so don't try using fakes or margarines. They don't work well for sautéing, and they can't deliver the wonderful taste of real butter.

However you cook it, seafood is an excellent choice for a lifetime of low-carb eating. With its abundant amounts of complete protein, you can enjoy it often.

Shrimp with Sun-Dried Tomatoes

Yield:	Serving size:	Prep time:	Cook time:
4 servings	¼ pound shrimp	15 minutes	12 to 15 minutes

Each serving has:			
7 g carbohydrate	2 g fiber	21 g protein	

1 garlic clove, minced

¼ cup butter (½ stick)

1 lb. large shrimp, peeled and deveined, about 33 shrimp

¼ cup sun-dried tomatoes, chopped

1 green bell pepper, cut into ½-in. pieces

1 (6.5-oz.) jar marinated artichoke hearts

½ cup pineapple, cut into chunks

1. Sauté garlic in butter in a large skillet.

2. Add shrimp, tomatoes, bell pepper, artichoke hearts, and pineapple. Cover and heat for 12 to 15 minutes until warm throughout.

RECIPE FOR SUCCESS

The combination of artichokes with crab and shrimp is a savory success. Baked like this, the dish can travel to potlucks or simply to the kitchen table. Serve with a side dish of salad or fruit.

Shrimp, Crab, and Artichokes au Gratin

Yield:	Serving size:	Prep time:	Cook time:
8 servings	¾ cup	30 minutes	30 minutes

Each serving has:			
3 g carbohydrate	2 g fiber	25 g protein	

¼ cup butter

½ lb. fresh white mushrooms, sliced

1 clove garlic, minced

2 TB. green onions, finely minced

1 TB. flour

½ tsp. fresh ground pepper

¾ cup heavy cream

8 oz. sharp cheddar cheese, grated, divided

½ cup dry white wine

2 (7.5-oz.) cans king crab, flaked and drained

1 lb. shrimp, cooked and peeled

1 (10-oz.) pkg. frozen artichoke hearts, cooked and drained

1. Preheat the oven to 375°F.

2. Melt butter in a skillet; add mushrooms, garlic, and green onions; sauté for 5 minutes.

3. Remove from heat and stir in flour, pepper, and cream. Slowly bring to a boil, stirring, and remove from heat. Add ½ cup cheese, and stir until melted. Stir in wine.

4. Combine sauce, crab, shrimp, artichokes, and 1 cup cheese. Pour into a buttered 2-quart casserole, and top with remaining ½ cup cheese.

5. Bake uncovered for 30 minutes or until bubbly and lightly browned.

Crab Cakes with Mustard Creole Sauce

Yield:	Serving size:	Prep time:	Cook time:
4 servings	1 cake	25 minutes	10 minutes

Each serving has:			
8 g carbohydrate	0 g fiber	21 g protein	

1 lb. fresh lump crabmeat

2 TB. green onions, finely chopped

1 TB. white wine

1 TB. plus 2 tsp. Dijon mustard

1 TB. lemon juice

3 TB. mayonnaise

White pepper to taste

1 egg white, slightly beaten

2 TB. finely crushed saltine crackers

1 TB. plus 1 TB. butter

¼ cup dry white vermouth or white wine

1 tsp. white wine vinegar

1 tsp. green onions, chopped

½ cup heavy cream

1 TB. red bell pepper, chopped and peeled

½ tsp. tarragon

Salt to taste

Cayenne to taste

Lemon wedges

1. To make crab cakes, combine crabmeat, green onions, white wine, 1 tablespoon Dijon mustard, lemon juice, mayonnaise, and white pepper in a bowl and mix gently. Add egg white and cracker crumbs to hold mixture together and mix gently. Shape into 4 patties.

2. In a skillet, heat 1 tablespoon of butter. Sauté crab cakes for 3 to 4 minutes on each side or until golden brown.

3. To make Mustard Creole Sauce, boil vermouth, vinegar, and green onions in a small, heavy saucepan until the mixture is reduced to 2 tablespoons. Add cream, red bell pepper, and tarragon. Boil until thickened and reduced to about ⅓ cup, stirring constantly.

4. Reduce the heat to medium-low. Whisk in vermouth-vinegar mixture and remaining 2 teaspoons Dijon mustard. Cook for 30 seconds. Whisk in remaining 1 tablespoon butter. Season with salt and cayenne. Keep warm until ready to serve. Serve crab cakes topped with Mustard Creole Sauce and lemon wedges.

RECIPE FOR SUCCESS

Tarragon makes every entrée taste special. Adding it to crab cakes, you have a down-home delight. Crab cakes are good hot or cold. Use leftovers—if there are any—for lunch and breakfast.

Crabmeat Florentine

Yield:	Serving size:	Prep time:	Cook time:
8 servings	¾ cup	20 minutes	45 minutes

Each serving has:		
4 g net carbohydrate	2 g fiber	13 g protein

4 (10-oz.) pkg. frozen spinach

2 TB. green onions, chopped

2 cloves garlic, minced

2 TB. plus 2 TB. butter (½ stick)

1 TB. flour

1 cup heavy cream

1 cup water

¼ cup white wine

Fresh parsley (to taste), chopped

2 TB. Parmesan cheese, grated

Salt and white pepper to taste

1 lb. lump crabmeat

1. Preheat the oven to 350°F.

2. Place spinach in a greased 3-quart casserole.

3. Sauté green onions and garlic in a small skillet with 2 tablespoons butter until onions are tender.

4. Melt remaining 2 tablespoons butter in a saucepan, stir in flour, and add cream and water gradually, stirring constantly. Cook until thickened, stirring constantly. Add wine, parsley, sautéed green onions, Parmesan cheese, salt, and pepper. Stir in crabmeat, and pour mixture over spinach.

5. Bake for 45 minutes or until bubbly.

DEFINITION

Florentine in a recipe usually means a savory main dish or side dish made with spinach. This recipe combines crab and spinach for a delectable main dish meal. Serve with a light side dish such as steamed vegetables or a raw fruit combination salad.

Crawfish Creole

Yield:	Serving size:	Prep time:	Cook time:
6 servings	1 cup	10 minutes	30 minutes

Each serving has:		
3 g carbohydrate	1 g fiber	21 g protein

1 medium onion, chopped	½ TB. cayenne
5 green onions, chopped	½ TB. white pepper
1 green bell pepper, chopped	1 lb. crawfish tails
½ cup butter (1 stick)	1 cup white wine
1 TB. Creole seasoning	1 cup heavy cream

1. Sauté onion, green onions, and bell pepper in butter in a skillet until onion is translucent. Add Creole seasoning, cayenne, and white pepper. Cook for 1 minute. Add crawfish tails and white wine. Simmer, covered, for 25 minutes.

2. Add cream and simmer for 5 minutes, stirring constantly.

Sautéed Shrimp in Artichoke Sauce

Yield:	Serving size:	Prep time:	Cook time:
4 servings	¼ pound shrimp with ¼ cup sauce	25 minutes	5 minutes

Each serving has:		
4 g carbohydrate	3 g fiber	23 g protein

1 lb. large shrimp (22–30 per lb.), peeled, deveined

1 TB. Creole seasoning

2 TB. plus 2 TB. butter (½ stick)

3 green onions, thinly sliced

2 (14-oz.) cans artichoke hearts, chopped and drained

½ cup dry white wine

1 cup heavy cream

Dash cayenne

Salt and freshly ground black pepper to taste

2 TB. fresh parsley, chopped

1. Sprinkle shrimp with Creole seasoning. Heat 2 tablespoons butter in a skillet over medium-high heat. Add shrimp and sauté until cooked. Remove shrimp and set aside.

2. Heat remaining 2 tablespoons butter in a skillet. Add green onions. Sauté until onions are soft but not brown. Add artichoke hearts and wine. Simmer for 5 minutes or until heated through. Stir in cream and season with cayenne, salt, and black pepper.

3. Arrange shrimp on individual serving plates. Spoon sauce over shrimp, and sprinkle with parsley.

RECIPE FOR SUCCESS

This recipe has a Southern taste with a beloved combination of artichokes and shrimp. To devein shrimp, remove the dark thread that runs up the back of the shrimp. The easiest way to do this is to make a cut with a small knife along the dark matter and then remove it.

Shrimp with Fennel and Green Beans

Yield:	Serving size:	Prep time:	Cook time:
4 servings	¼ pound shrimp	30 minutes	Included in prep time

Each serving has:		
1 g carbohydrate	1 g fiber	20 g protein

1 lb. large (22–30 per lb.) shrimp, peeled	½ tsp. dried parsley
4 TB. butter	½ cup fennel stalks, sliced
1 garlic clove, minced	1 cup green beans
	2 TB. sesame seeds

1. Sauté shrimp in butter with garlic and parsley 3 minutes or until shrimp begins to turn opaque. In a separate pan, steam fennel and green beans until tender.

2. Place shrimp in a serving dish, add fennel and green beans, and pour garlic butter sauce over all. Sprinkle with sesame seeds and serve warm.

RECIPE FOR SUCCESS

Fennel is similar to celery and grows with stalks and leaves. The seeds add great flavor to Italian dishes, and the stalks can be used like celery, as in this recipe. The taste is refreshing and slightly exotic. This unusual combination of tastes is quick and easy to prepare.

BBQ Shrimp

Yield:	Serving size:	Prep time:	Cook time:
6 servings	1/4 pound, approximately 1 dozen	5 minutes	25 minutes

Each serving has:		
2 g carbohydrate	< 1 g fiber	26 g protein

3 TB. butter	1 tsp. cayenne
1 large onion, chopped finely	1/4 cup Worcestershire sauce
1/2 cup celery, chopped	2 TB. steak sauce
1/2 cup Italian salad dressing	1 TB. lemon juice
1 TB. garlic, minced	3 lb. large (22–30 per lb.) shrimp, unpeeled
1 TB. paprika	
2 TB. freshly ground black pepper	

1. Melt butter in a cast-iron skillet or other heavy skillet, and sauté onion and celery until tender. Add Italian dressing, garlic, paprika, black pepper, cayenne, Worcestershire sauce, steak sauce, and lemon juice; stir well until it begins to boil. Add shrimp and simmer 15 minutes or until shrimp turn pink.

RECIPE FOR SUCCESS

"Real" BBQ shrimp is served in the shell and with rolls of paper towels—even newspaper has been seen as the tablecloth of choice! Die-hard seafood eaters even eat the shells. You can cheat a little and serve this delicious dish in a more civilized manner by peeling the shrimp before cooking—just be sure not to overcook. You will also need to reduce the amount of paprika, black pepper, and cayenne because you will not be seasoning through the shells. Without the peelings, you can eat the dish with a fork on good china and with cloth napkins!

Crab-Stuffed Eggplant

Yield:	Serving size:	Prep time:	Cook time:
6 servings	$\frac{1}{2}$ eggplant	10 minutes	1 hour

Each serving has:		
4 g carbohydrate	4 g fiber	17 g protein

3 medium-size eggplants	1 TB. lemon juice
3 TB. olive oil	1 TB. cornstarch
4 cloves garlic, minced	$\frac{1}{2}$ cup heavy cream
1 onion, chopped	1 tsp. white pepper
$\frac{1}{4}$ cup carrot, shredded	$\frac{1}{4}$ tsp. salt
3 TB. sliced celery	2 cups crabmeat
2 TB. fresh parsley, chopped	Paprika
Salt and pepper to taste	

1. Preheat the oven to 375°F. Butter a baking pan.

2. Cut eggplants in half lengthwise, and place cut side down onto the pan. Bake until eggplant is soft, about 35 minutes, and cool. Scoop out meat from eggplants and chop. Set shells aside.

3. Increase the oven temperature to 425°F. In a skillet, heat oil and sauté garlic, onion, carrot, celery, and parsley until vegetables are tender. Add chopped eggplant, salt, pepper, and lemon juice; cook 5 minutes.

4. Combine cornstarch, cream, white pepper, and salt; add to vegetable mixture, stirring constantly over low heat for 5 minutes until thickened and smooth.

5. Gently combine crabmeat with mixture, and spoon into eggplant shells. Place eggplant on a baking sheet, and sprinkle with paprika. Bake 15 to 20 minutes or until hot.

Crabmeat au Gratin

Yield:	Serving size:	Prep time:	Cook time:
8 servings	1 individual dish or approximately ½ cup	20 minutes	15 minutes

Each serving has:		
2 g carbohydrate	0 g fiber	23 g protein

2 TB. butter	1½ cups heavy cream
2 TB. fresh parsley, chopped	1 TB. sherry
¾ cup green onions, chopped	2 lb. lump crabmeat
1 TB. cornstarch	¾ cup (3-oz.) cheddar cheese, grated
½ tsp. dry mustard	

1. Preheat the oven to 375°F.

2. Melt butter in a pan over medium heat, and sauté parsley and green onions until tender.

3. Combine cornstarch and dry mustard, add cream, and stir until this makes a smooth paste. Slowly add this to onion mixture, and stir until smooth and thick. Remove from heat, and stir in sherry. Add crabmeat and mix gently.

4. Pour into individual serving dishes or one large baking dish. Sprinkle with cheese, and bake 15 minutes or until cheese is melted and bubbly.

Crawfish Étouffée

Yield:	Serving size:	Prep time:	Cook time:
8 servings	1 cup	30 minutes	30 minutes

Each serving has:		
5 g carbohydrate	1 g fiber	23 g protein

¼ cup butter (½ stick)

1 onion, chopped

1 bell pepper, chopped

½ cup celery, chopped

1 tsp. garlic, minced

¼ cup flour

1 tsp. cayenne

1 tsp. paprika

2 cups chicken broth or seafood stock

¼ cup fresh parsley, chopped

1 lb. crawfish tails, cooked and peeled or

1 lb. large shrimp, cooked and peeled, about 30

1. Melt butter in a large, heavy skillet, and sauté onion, bell pepper, celery, and garlic. Add flour, cayenne, and paprika, stirring constantly until brown, about 10 minutes. Be careful it does not stick or burn.

2. Add chicken broth and parsley, and stir until thick and simmering. Stir in crawfish or shrimp, and cook until heated through, about 5 minutes.

Variations: Traditionally, this wonderful dish is piled over white rice. Use lower-glycemic basmati rice or brown rice if you decide to use rice, and count the added carbohydrates. But, you can easily enjoy this *étouffée* without the rice. Étouffée seasonings and vegetable mixtures are sold in grocery stores and specialty food stores—just cook up a batch and freeze to have on hand to season any vegetable or meat dish. This saves you time because you don't have to chop and sauté each time you get ready to cook.

DEFINITION

Étouffée means smothered. But in today's lingo, expect étouffée to have a slightly browned butter and flour taste, which is very elegant and unusual.

Creamed Cajun Seafood

Yield:	Serving size:	Prep time:	Cook time:
6 servings	¾ cup	30 minutes	30 minutes
Each serving has:			
2 g carbohydrate	2 g fiber	15 g protein	

8 oz. pkg. cream cheese, cubed

3 TB. butter

1 lb. crawfish tails, cooked and peeled

½ cup onion, chopped

½ cup bell pepper, chopped

1 (8-oz.) pkg. fresh white mushrooms, coarsely chopped

1 TB. garlic powder

½ tsp. cayenne

1 cup heavy cream

1 cup Swiss cheese, grated

2 TB. sherry

½ cup pecans, chopped

1. Preheat the oven to 350°F.

2. In a double boiler over simmering water, melt cream cheese.

3. Melt butter in a skillet, and sauté crawfish tails, onion, bell pepper, mushrooms, garlic powder, and cayenne until vegetables are tender. Add cream, Swiss cheese, and sherry, stirring until cheese is melted and mixture is well combined.

4. Pour into a baking pan, and sprinkle pecans on top. Bake 30 minutes.

Variation: For a divine meal, use a grilled or baked fish fillet as a base, and top with a mixture of the shrimp or crawfish and lump crabmeat in the cream sauce.

Shrimp Scampi

Yield:	Serving size:	Prep time:	Cook time:
6 servings	1 dozen shrimp	10 minutes	15 minutes
Each serving has:			
3 g carbohydrate	0 g fiber	26 g protein	

¼ cup butter (½ stick)

¼ cup lemon juice

¼ cup green onions, chopped

2 TB. garlic, minced

1 TB. Worcestershire sauce

1 tsp. paprika

1 tsp. ground black pepper

2 drops hot sauce or ½ tsp. cayenne

6 dozen (22–30 per lb.) raw shrimp, peeled

1. In a large skillet or a Dutch oven, melt butter. Mix lemon juice, green onions, garlic, Worcestershire sauce, paprika, black pepper, and hot sauce into melted butter.

2. Add shrimp and stir to coat well. Stir and cook over medium heat until shrimp are pink. Watch closely so as not to overcook.

3. Serve with a side salad and green vegetable, like broccoli or green beans.

The Least You Need to Know

- Seafood meals are an excellent choice for low-carb eating.
- Today's grocery stores and fish markets offer a wide variety of fresh and frozen seafood year-round.
- Eat seafood steamed with drawn butter and lemon juice or in more elaborate dishes—either way seafood is a no-carb food.
- Seafood meals add variety to low-carb eating.

Fish Main Dishes

In This Chapter

- Enjoying meals from a vast selection of fish
- Benefiting from essential fats in cold-water fish
- Using new low-carb "breading" options

The vast variety of fish in the oceans and streams is astounding. Most of us have only eaten a few different kinds—salmon, tuna, halibut, and perhaps trout. Yet the oceans and streams have hundreds of edible species of fish, all with no carbohydrates. Even if you don't think of yourself as a fish eater, it's time you give fish a try.

Preparing fish is usually simple. But beware: plain fish can be rather boring and ordinary, which is exactly what you *don't* want when you are eating low carb. The recipes in this chapter can make fish not only interesting but also positively scrumptious! Grill fish, poach it, fry it, bake it, and then add seasonings and sauces that make it tasty and terrific.

Those Cold-Water Fish

Many of the recipes in this chapter call for cold-water fish, such as salmon, halibut, tuna, and trout. These varieties of fish deserve special mention because they contain nutrients that you need to be healthy.

These nutrients are called essential fatty acids, also known as EFAs. Eating just one serving a week can improve the health of your heart, reduce blood pressure, enhance moods, and improve brain function. In addition, they aid in the prevention of arthritis. Essential fatty acids aid in weight loss and weight management.

These fats, known as omega-3, 6, and 9 fatty acids, are deemed *essential* because you need to get them through your diet. Your body can't manufacture them by itself from other food you consume, as it can other fats.

> **DEFINITION**
>
> **Essential** is a term used by the government to designate a nutrient necessary to the body that has to be ingested or eaten. Your body can't manufacture an essential nutrient.

Fish Ingredients

Here are notes and ideas for ingredients used in these recipes.

- Some of the fish recipes call for using finely chopped nuts in place of the traditional breading. This dramatically reduces the number of carbohydrates in the dish and adds interesting flavors. To chop finely, process in a food processor or blender or hone your chopping skills with a chef's knife and chopping block.

- Use butter to grease a baking dish.

- Adding tangy, sweet, or savory ingredients is the key to making otherwise plain fish interesting to eat. In these recipes, you'll find macadamia nuts, lime juice, dill, tomatoes, black pepper, even olives, capers, and a mango salsa.

It's these other ingredients that bring fish to your palate in a pleasing and appetizing way. Eat a fish entrée at least once a week, and you'll get out of any low-carb eating rut you may be in.

Crispy Black Pepper Salmon

Yield:	Serving size:	Prep time:	Cook time:
4 servings	1 fillet	15 minutes plus 30 minutes marinating time	20 minutes

Each serving has:		
2 g carbohydrate	1 g fiber	37 g protein

½ cup dry white wine

¼ cup Worcestershire sauce

1 cup chicken broth

¼ tsp. salt

Dash white pepper

1 medium onion, peeled and very thinly sliced

4 (6-oz.) salmon fillets

2 TB. freshly cracked black pepper

2 TB. butter

1 bunch fresh spinach, washed, stemmed, and dried

1. In a resealable plastic bag, combine wine, Worcestershire sauce, chicken broth, salt, and white pepper. Add onion and salmon. Seal and chill at least 30 minutes.

2. Spread black pepper on a large plate. Remove salmon, reserving marinade and onion. Press both sides of salmon into pepper to coat and set aside. In a large skillet, heat butter over medium heat. Add onion to the skillet. Cook until onion is soft, about 5 minutes. Remove with a slotted spoon and set aside.

3. Increase heat to medium-high. Place salmon, flesh side down, in the skillet and cook until crisp and browned, about 4 minutes per side. When salmon is just cooked through, about 6 to 10 minutes, remove from the skillet.

4. Add spinach to the skillet, and cook until limp. Divide spinach equally among the plates. Cook marinade until reduced by ½, and divide equally over salmon.

RECIPE FOR SUCCESS

Salmon has a sturdy texture that can embrace the intense flavors of black pepper and spinach. With one vegetable serving in the spinach, this meal needs only a side salad or fruit to make a balanced meal.

Mediterranean Halibut

Yield:	Serving size:	Prep time:	Cook time:
8 servings	1 fillet	20 minutes	15 minutes
Each serving has:			
1 g carbohydrate	1 g fiber	21 g protein	

4 Italian plum tomatoes, seeded and diced

2 TB. Kalamata olives, chopped

$\frac{1}{4}$ cup drained capers

1 tsp. garlic, minced

2 TB. olive oil, divided

3 TB. fresh lemon juice, divided

$\frac{1}{4}$ cup dry white wine

$\frac{1}{4}$ cup crumbled feta cheese

2 TB. shallots, minced

2 TB. fresh basil, chopped

Salt and freshly ground black pepper

1 TB. butter

4 (6-oz.) halibut fillets

1. In a glass bowl, combine tomatoes, olives, capers, garlic, 2 tablespoons olive oil, $1\frac{1}{2}$ tablespoons lemon juice, wine, $\frac{1}{4}$ cup cheese, shallots, basil, salt, and pepper to taste.

2. Preheat the oven to 425°F. Grease the bottom of a shallow baking dish with butter. Season both sides of halibut with salt and pepper to taste. Place in the prepared baking dish. Squeeze remaining $1\frac{1}{2}$ tablespoons lemon juice over halibut and top with tomato mixture. Sprinkle with feta cheese.

3. Bake until just cooked through, about 15 minutes. Arrange halibut on individual serving plates and spoon pan juices on top.

Variation: You can substitute salmon, trout, red snapper, or any other sturdy fish for the halibut in this recipe.

RECIPE FOR SUCCESS

The Greek–Mediterranean flavors make this halibut dish interesting and delicious.

Red Snapper with Mango Salsa

Yield:	Serving size:	Prep time:	Cook time:
4 servings	1 fillet	25 minutes plus 30 minutes marinating time	20 minutes

Each serving has:		
7 g carbohydrate	1 g fiber	30 g protein

¼ cup plus 2 TB. fresh lime juice

2 TB. plus 3 TB. fresh cilantro, chopped

2 tsp. olive oil

4 (4-oz.) red snapper fillets

¼ tsp. plus ⅛ tsp. salt, divided

¼ tsp. plus ⅛ tsp. freshly ground black pepper

1 cup chopped Roma tomatoes, chopped

1 cup mango, chopped

1 TB. red onion, chopped

½ tsp. cumin

Dash hot sauce

1. To marinate red snapper, combine ¼ cup lime juice, 2 tablespoons cilantro, and olive oil in a large shallow dish and mix well. Place fish in marinade, turning to coat. Covered, marinate in the refrigerator for 30 minutes, turning once.

2. Drain fish and discard marinade. Sprinkle with ¼ teaspoon salt and ¼ teaspoon pepper. Place in a grilling basket. Grill over medium-hot (350°F–400°F) coals for 10 minutes on each side or until fish flakes easily. Place fish on a serving platter.

3. To make mango salsa, mix tomatoes, mango, red onion, 1 tablespoon cilantro, remaining ⅛ teaspoon salt and ⅛ teaspoon pepper, cumin, hot sauce, and remaining 2 tablespoons lime juice in a medium bowl.

4. Spoon mango salsa evenly over top of fish, and sprinkle with remaining 2 tablespoons cilantro.

RECIPE FOR SUCCESS

Fruit salsa is a healthful accompaniment to fish and can also count as one serving of fruits and vegetables for the day. This red snapper dish has a modern Southwest taste. The salsa contributes virtually all the carbohydrates in this dish, so you can cut your serving of the salsa in half and only get 9 grams carbohydrates.

Grilled Catfish with Mustard Sauce

Yield:	Serving size:	Prep time:	Cook time:
6 servings	1 fillet	15 minutes	10 minutes

Each serving has:		
4 g carbohydrate	0 g fiber	19 g protein

¼ cup onion, chopped

3 TB. butter

1 TB. flour

¼ tsp. dry mustard

1½ cups milk

1¼ cups shredded mild cheddar cheese

¾ cup white wine

1 TB. green onion, sliced

½ tsp. salt

¼ tsp. white pepper

6 (4-oz.) catfish fillets

1. In a large skillet, sauté onion in butter until translucent. Stir in flour and dry mustard. Cook for 1 minute, stirring constantly. Continue constant stirring as you add milk, and cook until thickened; add cheese and cook until cheese melts.

2. Add wine, green onion tops, salt, and white pepper; mix well.

3. Heat coals until gray or set dial on gas grill to medium-high temperature.

4. Place fish on the grill rack or in a greased fish basket. Grill for 5 to 8 minutes or until fish flakes easily. Serve with sauce.

RECIPE FOR SUCCESS

Catfish prepared any way at all is wonderful. And with this mustard sauce, it is deeply satisfying and interesting. A good tip for cooking fish is to measure its thickness; for best flavor it should be no more than 1 inch thick.

Five-Pepper Tuna

Yield:	Serving size:	Prep time:	Cook time:
6 servings	1 steak	15 minutes	10 minutes

Each serving has:		
0 g carbohydrate	0 g fiber	34 g protein

5 TB. five-pepper blend	$\frac{1}{4}$ cup cognac
6 (4-oz.) tuna steaks	$\frac{1}{2}$ cup chicken broth
Salt to taste	2 TB. Dijon mustard
2 TB. butter	1 cup heavy cream

1. Crush pepper blend, and spread on a plate or cutting board. Press tuna steaks into crushed pepper, turning to coat both sides. Sprinkle steaks with salt.

2. Melt butter in a sauté pan over high heat. Add steaks. Cook for 3 minutes on each side for rare or until steaks flake easily. Remove steaks to a warm platter.

3. Drain excess butter from the pan. Add cognac and cook over high heat, stirring to deglaze the pan. Add broth, mustard, and cream. Cook until sauce is reduced by $\frac{1}{2}$. Spoon sauce over tuna steaks and serve.

RECIPE FOR SUCCESS

The five-pepper blend, which can be purchased at a specialty food store, adds spicy heat, while the cream cools the palate. This is a different way to prepare fresh or frozen tuna.

Baked Salmon with Spinach Sauce

Yield:	Serving size:	Prep time:	Cook time:
8 servings	1 fillet	25 minutes	1 hour

Each serving has:		
1 g carbohydrate	0 g fiber	29 g protein

8 (4-oz.) salmon fillets

3 to 5 green onions, thinly sliced

1 lemon, thinly sliced

Salt and freshly ground black
    pepper to taste

$\frac{1}{2}$ cup spinach leaves

1 cup regular mayonnaise

1 to 2 TB. lemon juice

$\frac{1}{2}$ cup butter, melted

6 pieces of foil. Approximately
    12×8 inches

1. Preheat the oven to 350°F.

2. Lay each piece of salmon on a square piece of aluminum foil. Place some green onions and 1 lemon slice on each fillet. Sprinkle with salt and pepper to taste. Fold the foil around salmon, and fold the edges over to seal. Bake for 25 to 30 minutes.

3. While salmon is cooking, make sauce. Chop spinach in a food processor. Add mayonnaise and lemon juice, and process until blended. Melt butter and add slowly to spinach mixture until butter is thoroughly blended and sauce is thick.

4. Remove fillets from the oven. Unwrap the foil, remove salmon, and put on individual serving plates. Serve spinach sauce on the side.

Variation: Bake salmon with $\frac{1}{2}$ teaspoon dill and lemon slices.

RECIPE FOR SUCCESS

Baking the salmon in the foil "bag" keeps it very moist, tender, and tidy for cleanup. The sauce adds a nice tang to the salmon.

Pecan Trout

Yield:	Serving size:	Prep time:	Cook time:
6 servings	1 fillet	25 minutes	15 to 20 minutes

Each serving has:		
2 g carbohydrate	6 g fiber	30 g protein

2 cups pecan halves	$\frac{1}{4}$ tsp. salt
1 TB. flour	$\frac{1}{4}$ tsp. pepper
2 eggs	6 (3- to 4-oz.) trout fillets

1. Preheat the oven to 375°F.

2. In a food processor or blender, process $1\frac{1}{2}$ cups pecans until very finely chopped. Mix with flour, and put in a shallow pan.

3. Place remaining $\frac{1}{2}$ cup pecans in the microwave in a dish, and cook on high for 1 to 3 minutes until toasted.

4. Beat eggs with salt and pepper until blended. Dip each trout fillet into egg mixture and then into pecan mixture. Coat thoroughly and place in a buttered shallow baking dish. Bake for 15 to 20 minutes until trout is white and flakes.

5. Serve garnished with $\frac{1}{2}$ cup toasted pecan halves.

RECIPE FOR SUCCESS

Finely chopped pecans are a terrific substitute for breading on trout. Use freshly caught trout or purchase it from the fish section of the grocery store. The pecans keep the dish low carb compared to using flour or breading and add crunch plus flavor.

Tuna Fish Cakes

Yield:	Serving size:	Prep time:	Cook time:
4 servings	1 cake	10 minutes	8 minutes
Each serving has:			
1 g carbohydrate	0 g fiber	13 g protein	

1 egg
1 (6.5-oz.) can albacore tuna, drained
1 TB. green onions, chopped
2 TB. green pepper, chopped

3 TB. celery, chopped
¼ tsp. cayenne
Salt and pepper to taste
3 TB. butter
4 TB. grated Parmesan cheese

1. Beat egg slightly in a bowl. Add tuna, green onions, green pepper, celery, cayenne, salt, and pepper. Mix thoroughly.

2. Heat butter in a heavy skillet until melted and hot. Form tuna mixture into 4 cakes and place in skillet, cooking for 3 minutes per side. In the last minute, top each tuna cake with 1 tablespoon Parmesan cheese.

RECIPE FOR SUCCESS

This recipe makes a satisfying quick dinner. If dinner is on the run, add fresh apples and carrot sticks for a balanced meal. You can also make extra tuna fish cakes and keep them in the refrigerator to pack for lunch or eat for breakfast.

Salmon with Olives and Lemon

Yield:	Serving size:	Prep time:	Cook time:
5 servings	1 fillet	20 minutes	5 to 8 minutes
Each serving has:			
0 g carbohydrate	0 g fiber	21 g protein	

20-oz. salmon fillet
1 lemon
6 green olives stuffed with pimientos

Salt and freshly ground black pepper to taste
½ cup water

1. Preheat the oven to 500°F.

2. Place salmon on a foil-lined baking sheet. Cut lemon into ⅓-inch slices. Cut olives into ¼-inch slices. Place lemon and olive slices over salmon. Salt and pepper to taste. Pull up the sides of the foil and add water. Cover with foil, and seal the edges securely.

3. Oven "poach" salmon for 5 to 8 minutes or until cooked throughout so that the middle is not raw and is the same color as the outside of fish.

RECIPE FOR SUCCESS

This recipe gives a tangy Mediterranean taste to salmon. Cooking in the foil makes the salmon very tender and flaky. You can also grill the foil bag over high heat for 15 to 20 minutes.

Salmon with Macadamia Lime Butter

Yield:	Serving size:	Prep time:	Cook time:
4 servings	1 salmon steak	15 minutes	10 to 16 minutes

Each serving has:			
0 g carbohydrate	< 1 g fiber	36 g protein	

5 TB. butter	4 (5-oz.) salmon steaks
3 TB. lime juice	Salt and pepper to taste
2 TB. macadamia nuts, chopped	

1. To make butter sauce, melt butter in a small bowl in the microwave. Stir in lime juice and chopped macadamia nuts.

2. Season salmon steaks with salt and pepper. Cook salmon steaks on a gas or charcoal grill. Grill, covered, for 5 to 8 minutes per side until fish is cooked. Remove to a serving platter, and top with butter sauce.

TABLE TALK

This dish scores a home run. Quick and easy to prepare, the mixture of lime, butter, and macadamia nuts makes this salmon dish appealing to eaters of all ages. Use nut flour or ground nuts for breading on fish and meats. It actually adds more flavor than regular breading made with wheat, while it lowers the carb count and the glycemic index of the food. Plus, the nuts contain more nutrients.

Blackened Fish

Yield:	Serving size:	Prep time:	Cook time:
6 servings	1 fillet	5 minutes plus time to prepare spice mixture	5 minutes

Each serving has:			
1 g carbohydrate	0 g fiber	30 g protein	

2 tsp. onion powder

2 tsp. cayenne

1 tsp. freshly ground black pepper

1 tsp. thyme

1 TB. garlic powder

1 TB. paprika

1 tsp. salt

1 tsp. white pepper

1 tsp. oregano

1 pinch sage

2 TB. butter, unmelted, plus 2 TB. butter, melted, divided

6 (5-oz.) fish fillets

Lemon wedges for serving

1. Combine onion powder, cayenne, black pepper, thyme, garlic powder, paprika, salt, white pepper, oregano, and sage to create the Cajun Spice Mix. Store extra in a sealed jar in the refrigerator. Use the mixture in other Cajun recipes or anytime a spicy taste is desired.

2. Wash fish and pat dry. Coat each side with melted butter, and sprinkle Cajun spice liberally on both sides.

3. In a cast-iron skillet, heat butter over high heat to just short of smoking. Cook fish 1 minute until the side down begins to char, quickly flip fish over, and cook the other side in the same manner.

4. Serve with lemon wedges.

RECIPE FOR SUCCESS

The Cajun Spice Mix is just as delicious when used to season grilled, baked, or pan-fried fish. Serve with Southern Greens or Creamed Cabbage (see recipe in Chapter 19), Cajun Dirty Rice (see recipe in Chapter 23), Minty Fruit (see recipe in Chapter 21), and your favorite dessert. Each tablespoon equals 1 gram carbohydrate.

HOT POTATO

The cast-iron skillet has to be almost white hot for the fish to blacken and not burn. The blackening process happens quickly and may produce a lot of smoke. Some folks prefer to use this method of cooking outdoors on a fish cooker.

Salmon in Dill Sauce

Yield:	Serving size:	Prep time:	Cook time:
6 servings	1 steak with ¼ cup sauce	15 minutes	8 minutes

Each serving has:		
4 g carbohydrate	0 g fiber	25 g protein

2 tsp. dried dill weed or 2 TB. fresh
dill weed, chopped

½ tsp. white pepper

2 TB. spicy prepared mustard

1 TB. white wine vinegar

1 tsp. honey

1 cup plain yogurt, such as Greek
yogurt

2 TB. red onion, finely chopped

6 (4-oz.) salmon steaks

Olive oil

1. Combine dill, white pepper, mustard, vinegar, honey, yogurt, and onion. Refrigerate until ready to serve.

2. Heat grill. Brush salmon steaks with olive oil and grill 5 to 8 minutes per side, depending on thickness of steaks.

3. Place salmon on serving platter, and top each with Dill Sauce. Save any leftover sauce for use later.

RECIPE FOR SUCCESS

The Dill Sauce is delicious as a vegetable dip or salad dressing. You can also refrigerate the salmon and serve it cold over fresh baby spinach leaves. If desired, poach or bake the salmon instead of grilling it. It is delicious cooked by any method, and leftover salmon makes the perfect breakfast protein.

Trout Dinner in a Bag

Yield:	Serving size:	Prep time:	Cook time:
6 servings	1 fillet with 1 cup vegetables	15 minutes	30 minutes

Each serving has:		
10 g carbohydrate	5 g fiber	30 g protein

½ cup green onion, chopped

1 tsp. white pepper

6 (4-oz.) trout fillets (or use any fish desired)

1 lb. fresh or frozen whole green beans

3 medium turnips, peeled and sliced

6 carrots, shredded or chopped

6 TB. butter

6 sprigs fresh parsley

1. Preheat the oven to 350°F.

2. In a small bowl, combine green onion and pepper and set aside.

3. Put a large baking bag in a baking pan. Place fillets, green beans, turnips, and carrots in the bottom of the bag. Sprinkle with onion-pepper mixture; top each fillet with 1 tablespoon butter and 1 sprig parsley. Close the bag, and cut vent holes according to manufacturer's directions. Bake for 30 minutes until fish flakes and vegetables are tender.

Variation: As an alternative to a cooking bag, you can place each fillet and ⅙ of all ingredients into individual sheets of aluminum foil. Fold into foil packets and serve them on plates. This basic recipe is delicious when using poultry in place of the fish; increase cooking time accordingly for the poultry.

The Least You Need to Know

- Fish is a wise nutritional choice for low-carb eating.
- The varieties of fish are endless, and the tastes, diverse and interesting.
- Use marinating and nut coatings to make tasty fish main dishes.
- Cold-water fish contain essential fatty acids you need for a strong body, a healthy heart, and weight loss.

Main Dish Combinations

The combination of ingredients—proteins, fats, and vegetables—prepared and cooked together delivers great food and eating value. Here are recipes for timesaving one-pot meals, plus soups and stews. They feature your favorite meats and ingredients.

Eggs and cheese blend well together to deliver creamy entrées complemented with vegetables, herbs, and spices. Main dish salads meet your highest expectations for interesting tastes and textures.

One-Pot Meals

Chapter 13

In This Chapter

- Slow cooking with the oven, stove, or slow cooker
- Converting recipes for the slow cooker
- A convenient balanced meal in a pot

Casseroles are back in popularity but under a different name—one-pot meals. Just toss delicious low-carb ingredients into a baking dish, Dutch oven, or slow cooker; return sometime between 2 to 8 hours later; and voilà—dinner is ready.

We know your lifestyle is busy. You rush to keep up with multiple demands at work, at home, and even at play. You want to eat low carb, yet fast food beckons at every corner. One-pot meals let you add some stability and order into your day and your eating. Best of all, you can easily make your one-pot meals low carb and totally scrumptious.

Your Choice of Cookware

One-pot cooking requires different kinds of cookware. Our recipes use the following types:

- **Oven casserole.** Use a glass or enameled baking dish. Some recipes require a lid. You can put the pot in the oven before you leave for work or play.
- **Dutch oven.** Usually made from cast iron, the Dutch oven is used for top-of-the-stove cooking. The cast iron evenly distributes heat and is ideal for low-temperature simmering.

- **Slow cooker.** This electrical appliance cooks at a very low temperature. It may take 4 to 8 hours to cook a pot roast, but it is ideal for when you will be away from home for hours. It uses very little electricity, and the newer models clean up easily, as the crockery cooking chamber comes out and can go into the dishwasher. Don't lift the lid on your slow cooker during cooking. Every time you do, it can take the pot 20 minutes to return to its previous cooking temperature.

With one-pot meals, you cook vegetables and meat together so you get both complete protein and at least one vegetable and often two—a balanced and nutritious meal. You can serve each of these recipes by itself or add one more vegetable or salad as a side dish if you prefer. These vegetable and meat combinations are low carb and are hearty enough to serve you and your entire family.

Adapting for the Slow Cooker

You can adapt any of these recipes to cook in the slow cooker. Just follow these guidelines:

- **Vegetables.** Dense vegetables like carrots and other root vegetables should be cut no larger than 1-inch thick and placed in the bottom of the pot because they take longer to cook. Other vegetables, such as tomatoes and parsley, can be put on top of the meat or mixed in with it.

- **Liquids.** Decrease the quantity of liquids in slow cooking to about half the recipe's recommended amount. One cup liquid is usually plenty.

- **Herbs and spices.** Whole herbs release flavors over time, so they are a good choice for slow cooking. Ground herbs and spices lose pungency when slow cooked, so add them near the end of cooking, about an hour before serving. As in all cooking, taste and adjust seasonings, if necessary, before serving.

- **Milk/cheese.** Add these during the last hour, as they don't hold up well during slow cooking.

- **Preparation.** Browning meats first in a heavy skillet can enhance flavor. This also decreases the amount of fat in the food. For a special taste treat, after browning, deglaze the skillet with wine, a little vinegar, lemon, or broth, and add the liquid to the pot.

Follow this time guide for converting regular one-pot recipes for the slow cooker.

Conventional Recipe	Low (200°F)	High (300°F)
15 to 30 minutes	4 to 6 hours	1½ to 2 hours
35 to 45 minutes	6 to 10 hours	3 to 4 hours
50 minutes to 3 hours	8 to 18 hours	4 to 6 hours

One-Pot Ingredients

One-pot recipes lend themselves to the use of almost any ingredient imaginable. Fresh ingredients are best, of course, as they contain more nutrients, but because everything is cooked all together, you can often use canned ingredients and not notice much difference in taste.

Meat and Cheese Loaf

Yield:	Serving size:	Prep time:	Cook time:
12 servings	1 slice	20 minutes	1½ hours
Each serving has:			
5 g carbohydrate	1 g fiber	29 g protein	

2 lb. ground beef chuck

1 cup Swiss cheese, grated

2 large eggs, lightly beaten

½ cup onion, chopped

½ cup green pepper, chopped

1½ tsp. salt

½ tsp. freshly ground black pepper

1 tsp. celery salt

2 cups milk

¼ cup dry breadcrumbs

4 slices lean bacon

1. Preheat the oven to 350°F.

2. Mix together beef, Swiss cheese, eggs, onion, green pepper, salt, black pepper, celery salt, milk, and breadcrumbs. Pack into a large loaf pan or 2 smaller loaf pans. Top with bacon and bake 1 to 1½ hours. Cool for 5 minutes, and slice loaf into 12 portions.

RECIPE FOR SUCCESS

This recipe is a variation on meat loaf—both cheese and meat in a loaf. Prepare enough for one meal, and use the leftovers for lunch and dinner. Good side dishes include green vegetables such as broccoli, spinach, green peas, and green beans.

Braised Beef with Italian Herbs

Yield:	Serving size:	Prep time:	Cook time:
8 servings	4 ounces	20 minutes	1½ to 2 hours

Each serving has:		
3 g carbohydrate	0 g fiber	43 g protein

¼ cup butter (½ stick)

3 lb. rump or chuck roast

1 cup beef broth or water

1 small onion, minced

1 clove garlic, minced

1 small carrot, minced

1 stalk celery, minced

1 cup tomatoes, chopped

½ tsp. dried oregano

½ tsp. dried rosemary

2 whole cloves

1 cup red wine

1. Heat butter in a Dutch oven or heavy saucepan with a tight-fitting lid.

2. Brown meat well on all sides over medium heat for about 15 to 20 minutes. Add beef broth, onion, garlic, carrot, celery, tomatoes, oregano, rosemary, cloves, and wine. Simmer over low heat 1½ to 2½ hours or until meat is tender.

3. Remove meat to a serving platter. Slice meat into 8 servings. Prepare this recipe 1 day ahead of time or freeze.

Variation: You can make this in a slow cooker by putting all ingredients except the butter directly into the slow cooker and cooking on high for 6 to 7 hours.

Beef Ratatouille Pie

Yield:	Serving size:	Prep time:	Cook time:
8 servings	1 wedge	30 minutes	45 minutes

Each serving has:			
8 g carbohydrate	5 g fiber	24 g protein	

1½ lb. extra-lean ground beef	2 small green bell peppers, cored, seeded, and thinly sliced
½ cup red bell pepper, chopped	1 tsp. garlic, minced
1 cup tomato sauce	½ lb. ripe tomatoes, chopped
½ tsp. dried oregano	1½ tsp. dried basil
3 tsp. salt	½ cup fresh parsley leaves, minced
¼ tsp. freshly ground black pepper	1 medium eggplant, quartered and thinly sliced
2 TB. butter	2 small zucchini, thinly sliced
1 large yellow onion, peeled, quartered, and sliced	2 small yellow squash, thinly sliced
1 large red onion, peeled, quartered, and sliced	1 tsp. dried thyme, crumbled

1. Preheat the oven to 350°F.

2. In a large bowl, combine beef, red bell pepper, ½ cup tomato sauce, oregano, 1 teaspoon salt, and pepper. Press into bottom and sides of a 10-inch deep-dish pie pan. Bake 20 minutes. Remove from the oven, leaving the oven on. Drain and set aside.

3. In a large skillet, heat 1 tablespoon butter over high heat. Add yellow and red onions and green bell peppers, and cook just until soft. Stir in garlic, tomatoes, and remaining ½ cup tomato sauce. Cover, reduce heat to medium, and cook 5 minutes. Remove cover and cook until juices have evaporated. Add basil and parsley.

4. In a large bowl, sprinkle eggplant, zucchini, and yellow squash with remaining 2 teaspoons salt. Let stand 30 minutes to release moisture and then pat dry. In a skillet with a lid, heat remaining 1 tablespoon butter over high heat. Add eggplant, zucchini, and yellow squash, and cook 3 minutes. Stir in thyme.

5. Spread about ¹⁄₃ tomato mixture evenly over prepared meat shell. Cover with ¹⁄₂ eggplant mixture. Add another ¹⁄₃ tomato mixture, and cover with remaining eggplant mixture. Top with remaining tomato mixture. Cover with foil and bake 25 minutes. Remove the foil and continue baking 20 minutes. Cut into 8 wedges before serving.

RECIPE FOR SUCCESS

This is a complete balanced meal as it is. You get complete protein from the meat and plenty of vegetables. The higher carbs come from the vegetables in the pie. Plus, it tastes great.

Veal Italian Style

Yield: 6 servings	Serving size: ¾ cup	Prep time: 25 minutes	Cook time: 1 hour
Each serving has: 2 g carbohydrate	0 g fiber	28 g protein	

¼ cup butter (½ stick)	¼ tsp. dried rosemary
2 lb. boneless veal, cut into 1-in. cubes	¼ tsp. dried oregano
1 medium onion, chopped	½ tsp. salt
2 stalks celery, cut into 1-in. pieces	¼ tsp. fresh ground pepper
2 cups fresh mushrooms, sliced	1 cup dry white wine

1. Preheat the oven to 350°F.

2. Melt butter in a casserole on the stove. Add veal and brown on all sides for 10 minutes. Add onion, celery, and mushrooms; sauté 5 minutes. Add rosemary, oregano, salt, pepper, and wine. Cover and bake for 1 hour, stirring occasionally.

RECIPE FOR SUCCESS

This recipe adds the taste and aroma of Italian cooking without any high-carb pasta. If you prefer, substitute 1 cup water plus 1 teaspoon vinegar for the wine. The wine or vinegar helps tenderize the meat as it cooks, and this small amount doesn't change the taste of the recipe. You can also cook this in a slow cooker on low for 4 to 6 hours. Serve with puréed cauliflower and Fennel and Tomatoes (see recipe in Chapter 19).

Peppered Tenderloin Casserole

Yield:	Serving size:	Prep time:	Cook time:
6 servings	¾ cup	30 minutes	30 minutes

Each serving has:			
7 g carbohydrate	2 g fiber	35 g protein	

4 TB. butter

2 lb. beef tenderloin or boneless sirloin, cut into ¼-in. strips

1 tsp. salt

½ tsp. black pepper

⅛ tsp. dried sage

⅛ tsp. dried cumin

2 cups quartered mushrooms

2 cloves garlic, minced

1 medium onion, chopped

1 green pepper, sliced

1 red pepper, sliced

2 celery stalks, chopped

2 tomatoes, cut into wedges

¼ cup soy sauce

2 TB. apple cider vinegar

2 TB. tomato paste

1. Preheat the oven to 325°F.

2. Heat 2 tablespoons butter in a heavy skillet, and quickly brown beef on all sides. Put beef into a 4-quart casserole. Sprinkle with salt, pepper, sage, and cumin, and stir to mix.

3. Sauté mushrooms in remaining 2 tablespoons butter. Add garlic, onion, green and red peppers, and celery. Sauté for an additional 3 minutes. Put mixture into the casserole and add tomatoes.

4. Put soy sauce, vinegar, and tomato paste into the skillet and cook, stirring to loosen browned particles. Pour over meat and vegetables in the casserole. Toss lightly to mix.

5. Bake 30 minutes or until meat is tender and mixture is bubbling.

 RECIPE FOR SUCCESS

Great for serving a crowd or for a potluck dinner, this casserole has the flavor of fajitas in one pot. Serve it all by itself or with guacamole or avocado salad.

Basil Pot Roast

Yield:	Serving size:	Prep time:	Cook time:
8 servings	4 ounces beef with 1 carrot and ½ cup cauliflower	15 minutes	2½ to 3 hours

Each serving has:		
9 g carbohydrate	4 g fiber	31 g protein

1 (3-lb.) pot roast

2 TB. olive oil or butter

1 (16-oz.) can tomato sauce

½ cup red wine

2 medium onions, chopped

5 cloves garlic, minced

1 TB. freshly ground black pepper

4 TB. fresh basil or 2 TB. dried

1 tsp. dried oregano

1 cup beef broth

6 large carrots, cut in half

1. Preheat the oven to 350°F.

2. In a Dutch oven, brown roast on all sides in hot oil.

3. To make sauce, combine tomato sauce, red wine, onions, garlic, black pepper, basil, oregano, and beef broth. Pour over meat in the pot and cover. Bake 2½ to 3 hours until roast is tender.

4. Add carrots the last 40 minutes of baking time.

RECIPE FOR SUCCESS

The gravy is delicious served over mashed cauliflower instead of potatoes. By itself, this is a complete balanced meal, as you have the carrots and cauliflower for vegetables. If you like, add a fruit salad for something light with the meal.

Slow Cooker Italian Brisket

Yield:	Serving size:	Prep time:	Cook time:
8 servings	4 oz. brisket	15 minutes	11 hours
Each serving has:			
5 g carbohydrate	0 g fiber	30 g protein	

1 (2- to 3-lb.) boneless brisket

2 cups spaghetti sauce (purchased or homemade)

2 medium onions, chopped

1 bell pepper, chopped

1 TB. molasses

$\frac{1}{2}$ tsp. Italian seasoning

$\frac{1}{4}$ tsp. cayenne

2 TB. Worcestershire sauce

1$\frac{1}{2}$ cups shredded white cheese (mozzarella, Swiss, provolone, Parmesan, etc.)

1. Thinly slice beef diagonally across the grain. In a bowl, combine spaghetti sauce with onions, bell pepper, molasses, Italian seasoning, cayenne, and Worcestershire sauce. Place beef in a slow cooker, and cover with seasoned sauce. Cover and cook on high for first hour; turn to low for 10 hours. Serve with shredded cheese on top.

HOT POTATO

It is easier to slice raw beef when it is partially frozen. Use this technique when you need slices for stir-fry or fajitas.

RECIPE FOR SUCCESS

Put together this recipe the day before and add to the slow cooker early in the morning to be ready for supper. Or if you prefer to cook ahead and just reheat, add it to the slow cooker to reheat 2 to 3 hours before serving time. Use 1 slice Low-Carb Bread for a wonderful open-face Italian sandwich; remember to add additional carbohydrates. Serve with Five-Day Coleslaw (see recipe in Chapter 20) and Chocolate Mousse (see recipe in Chapter 25) for dessert.

Eggplant and Meat Casserole

Yield:	Serving size:	Prep time:	Cook time:
6 servings	1/6 recipe	15 minutes	30 minutes

Each serving has:		
11 g carbohydrate	8 g fiber	29 g protein

1 lb. ground beef

1 (16-oz.) can tomato sauce

1/4 cup Italian seasoned
  breadcrumbs

2 TB. Parmesan cheese

1 tsp. dried oregano

2 eggplants

3 large egg whites, slightly beaten

1 cup mozzarella cheese, shredded

1. Preheat the oven to 350°F.

2. In a heavy skillet, brown beef and drain. Mix in tomato sauce and set aside.

3. Combine breadcrumbs, Parmesan cheese, and oregano and set aside.

4. Peel eggplants and slice lengthwise into thin lasagna-like strips, about 1/8 inch.
   Dip eggplant in egg whites and then into breadcrumb mixture. Bake slices on a
   baking sheet for 20 minutes.

5. In a buttered oblong baking dish, layer eggplant "noodles," 1/3 beef mixture, and
   1/3 mozzarella cheese mixture; repeat layers until all ingredients are used. Bake
   10 minutes or until cheese melts and lasagna is bubbling. Slice into 6 servings.

Jambalaya

Yield:	Serving size:	Prep time:	Cook time:
8 servings	1 cup	20 minutes	15 minutes plus time to prepare shrimp

Each serving has:			
15 g carbohydrate	2 g fiber	26 g protein	

2 chicken bouillon cubes

1½ cups boiling water

2 TB. butter

2 medium onions, chopped

1 bell pepper, chopped

¼ cup celery, chopped

½ cup raw basmati rice

1 (28-oz.) can whole tomatoes, cut in quarters

1½ tsp. Cajun Spice Mix (see Chapter 12)

2 lb. large shrimp (about 60), cooked, peeled, and chopped

¼ cup green onions, finely chopped for garnish

1. Dissolve chicken bouillon cubes in boiling water and set aside.

2. In a Dutch oven, melt butter and sauté onions, bell pepper, and celery until tender. Add chicken bouillon and raw rice; simmer 15 minutes. Add tomatoes and Cajun Spice Mix, and simmer 5 minutes until rice is done. Add shrimp and simmer just until heated.

3. Serve garnished with green onions.

RECIPE FOR SUCCESS

Any seafood or mixture may be substituted for shrimp. Chicken with sausage makes a great jambalaya as well. Rice is included in this dish and adds 11 carbs per serving. Omit the rice and only use 1 cup water if you want to have fewer carbs. The carb count without the rice is 19 grams per serving. Serve with a large mixed green salad.

Stewed Chicken

Yield:	Serving size:	Prep time:	Cook time:
6 servings	4 ounces	10 minutes in slow cooker	3 to 10 hours

Each serving has:			
3 g carbohydrate	1 g fiber	28 g protein	

1 whole chicken	$\frac{1}{2}$ tsp. salt
1 TB. garlic powder	2 TB. Worcestershire sauce
2 TB. dried parsley	$\frac{1}{4}$ cup water
$\frac{1}{2}$ tsp. cayenne	3 onions, halved
$\frac{1}{2}$ tsp. freshly ground black pepper	

1. Wash and dry chicken, removing and discarding neck and giblets from cavity. Mix together garlic powder, parsley, cayenne, black pepper, and salt. Season inside cavity with spices and Worcestershire sauce. Pour water into a slow cooker, and place chicken inside the pot. Lay onion pieces around chicken and cover. Cook on low 10 hours or high for 3 hours.

2. Serve immediately or refrigerate separately from broth to use later.

RECIPE FOR SUCCESS

This is such an easy way to get de-boned chicken for recipes. The meat just falls off the bone. Refrigerate the chicken and de-bone the next day, and chill the broth and remove congealed fat the next day. Thicken broth for gravy or use as stock for recipes. Freeze broth in ice cube trays and use for seasoning as needed.

Your Choice Stir-Fry

Yield:	**Serving size:**	**Prep time:**	**Cook time:**
6 servings	3 ounces meat, 2½ cups vegetables	30 minutes	15 minutes

Each serving has:		
2 g carbohydrate	7 g fiber	25 g protein

Protein	Veggie A	Veggie B	Crunch	Necessities
1 lb. beef top round, partially frozen and thinly sliced	1 cup broccoli florets	1 cup fresh mushrooms, thinly sliced	1 cup walnut pieces	⅓ cup water; 2 tsp. cornstarch
1 lb. boneless pork, partially frozen and thinly sliced	1 cup fresh asparagus, cut into 1-in. lengths	2 cups chopped Chinese cabbage	1 cup dry-roasted peanuts	2 TB. soy sauce; 1 TB. dry sherry (or bouillon granules and water)
2 whole large boneless chicken breasts, skinned	2 large carrots, halved lengthwise	2 stalks celery, thinly sliced	1 cup pea pods, thinly bias sliced 4 green onions, thinly sliced	2 TB. oil; 1 clove garlic, minced; and cut into 1-in. pieces
1 lb. medium shrimp, peeled and deveined	½ cup cauliflower florets, thinly sliced	2 medium tomatoes, cut into wedges and seeded	1 (8-oz.) can sliced water chestnuts, drained	½ cup bean sprouts or bamboo shoots, no liquid

1. Choose ingredients from each of the first four columns. Use all ingredients in the last column, *Necessities*, in every recipe. Prepare all ingredients as needed before the cooking begins.

2. Combine water, cornstarch, soy sauce, and sherry, and set aside.

3. In a covered saucepan, cook *Veggie A* in boiling salted water for 3 minutes. Drain well and set aside.

4. In a large wok or a skillet, heat oil and stir-fry garlic and green onions. Add *Crunch* ingredient and bean sprouts. Stir-fry 1 to 2 minutes. Remove from the pan and set aside.

5. Add more oil, if needed. Add $\frac{1}{2}$ *Protein* choice, and stir-fry 2 to 3 minutes or until browned. Remove from the pan and set aside while cooking remaining *Protein* choice. Return all *Protein* food to the pan, and add *Crunch* ingredient mixture.

6. Stir in soy sauce mixture, and cook until thickened and bubbly. Stir in *Veggies A* and *B;* cover and heat 1 minute.

RECIPE FOR SUCCESS

With this recipe, you can have stir-fry for days and never end up with the same combo! Mix and match additional great veggies such as bell pepper, red onion, or brussels sprouts; vary the nuts and add sesame seeds. A great party idea is to have guests choose their own ingredients and cook in separate electric woks or skillets. Add additional carbohydrate if served over rice.

The Least You Need to Know

- One-pot meals give you ultimate convenience and low-carb eating.
- Cook one-pot meals when you are away from home for a while, simply relaxing, or too busy to be in the kitchen.
- Give one-pot meals flavor and aroma variety with international or regional flavors.
- One-pot meals give you a nutritionally balanced meal.
- You can convert any one-pot meal for cooking in the slow cooker.

Low-Carb Soups and Stews

In This Chapter

- Cooking comfort food like Mother's chicken soup
- Varying your standard noodle soup
- Boosting your immune system

For many of us, when the weather turns cold and damp, soups and stews offer both comfort and nutrition. They ward off the damp. They overcome the chill in our bodies. They warm our hands and mouth and seem to heat our whole insides.

Maybe it's the pleasure that comes from slurping up a liquid-based dish, but eating soups and stews seems to evoke feelings of an earlier time and causes us to remember Mama's nurturing cooking. They seem to nurture the whole body. And yes, chicken soup really is good for what ails you!

A good soup is special. A cup of something delicious at the start of a meal delights the palate. A whole bowl of a hearty soup can serve as a meal in itself. A stew seems ideal for a winter evening when you want to keep the cold outside while you, your family, and your friends warm your insides inside!

Ladle the Soup, Hold the Noodles

Traditional soups and stews often have noodles, rice, or potatoes, but these ingredients aren't at all necessary to taste or warmth. The recipes in this chapter give soups and stews a distinctly modern twist. So don't expect to find many starchy foods. Just forget about those starches! You don't need them.

These recipes add more of what your body needs and actually yearns for. What's that? More vegetables that support you in health and help you with weight management. But the rich taste remains with the use of such ingredients as heavy cream, cheese, and legumes.

As you and your body get accustomed to the succulent and hearty taste of these soups and stews, you'll prefer leaving out the high-carbohydrate starches.

Good for What Ails You

Nothing soothes the yucky feeling of a cold like a bowl of chicken soup. Scientists have actually figured out why. Chicken soup has anti-inflammatory properties and boosts the immune system. The soup also helps stop the movement of neutrophils, which are cells that are released in the presence of viral infections such as colds and flu and result in increased mucus production. Thus, soup helps dry up your runny nose.

In this chapter, you find an old-country recipe for chicken soup and a quite modern one for tortilla soup, also made with chicken. But you don't need to have a cold or the flu to enjoy these soups and stews. They're wonderful any time.

TABLE TALK

Serve soups and stews for any meal. Yes, they taste great for lunch, but what about breakfast? A hearty soup or stew may be just the right breakfast before a day of skiing, snowshoeing, or hiking. They can even be just the right thing before school or before work. You don't need to limit your breakfast eating to the standard expected fare. Perk up your day and the days of your loved ones with soups and stews—all of which are low-carb, of course.

Beef Soup with Vegetables

Yield:	Serving size:	Prep time:	Cook time:
10 servings	1 cup	30 minutes	3 hours

Each serving has:		
4 g carbohydrate	2 g fiber	30 g protein

2 lb. beef brisket, cut into chunks	$\frac{1}{2}$ cup spinach
1 carrot	$\frac{1}{2}$ cup peas
$\frac{1}{2}$ head cabbage	1 (14.5-oz.) can tomatoes
3 spears asparagus	1 bay leaf
1 stalk celery	1 pinch dried thyme
1 small bunch parsley	1 pinch dried oregano
1 small onion	Salt and freshly ground black pepper to taste
$\frac{1}{2}$ cup string beans	

1. Put beef in a large pot or a Dutch oven. Cover with cold water, and boil for $\frac{1}{2}$ hour. During this time, cut carrot, cabbage, asparagus, celery, parsley, onion, string beans, and spinach into 1-inch chunks.

2. Skim the pot carefully, then add all cut vegetables plus peas, tomatoes, bay leaf, thyme, and oregano. Add salt and pepper to taste.

3. Simmer very slowly for 3 hours. Remove bay leaf. Serve with horseradish for meat.

HOT POTATO

Be sure to check the pot about every half hour to make sure it is simmering enough but not boiling. You may need to add water from time to time to keep the water level high enough to cook the vegetables.

Mexican Meat Soup

Yield:	Serving size:	Prep time:	Cook time:
8 servings	¾ cup	20 minutes	1 hour

Each serving has:		
4 g carbohydrate	< 1 g fiber	31 g protein

2 lb. round steak, cut into cubes

1 lb. pork shoulder, cut into cubes

3 TB. butter

1 (4-oz.) can green chilies, diced

3 green onions, chopped

3 sprigs mint

½ tsp. garlic, minced

¼ cup fresh parsley, chopped

1 pinch cumin

½ tsp. ground cloves

6 cups water

1 cup tomato juice

Salt and freshly ground black pepper to taste

1. Brown steak and pork in butter, and add chilies, onions, mint, garlic, parsley, cumin, and cloves into a large pot with a lid. Add water, tomato juice, salt, and pepper to taste. Cover tightly and simmer for 1 hour.

Mexican Chicken Avocado Soup

Yield:	Serving size:	Prep time:	Cook time:
6 servings	1 cup	25 minutes	15 minutes

Each serving has:		
6 g carbohydrate	3 g fiber	15 g protein

1 TB. olive oil

1 small onion, coarsely chopped

2 large garlic cloves, minced

1 TB. chili powder

2 tsp. cumin

½ tsp. dried oregano

6 cups chicken stock

1 medium tomato, diced

1½ tsp. salt

¼ tsp. freshly ground black pepper

1 large chicken breast

½ cup frozen corn

1 avocado, sliced

1. Heat olive oil in a skillet. Add onion and sauté until onion is translucent. Add garlic, chili powder, cumin, and oregano. Sauté for 1 minute.

2. Add chicken stock, diced tomato, salt, and pepper. Bring to a boil. Add chicken. Simmer, covered, about 15 minutes or until chicken is cooked through. Remove chicken to a plate and cool slightly.

3. Shred chicken, discarding skin and bones. Add corn to soup. Simmer until corn is tender. Add shredded chicken. Simmer for 1 minute. Ladle into soup bowls. Top with avocado slices. *Note:* You can prepare soup 1 to 3 days in advance.

4. Chill, covered, in the refrigerator and reheat before serving.

RECIPE FOR SUCCESS

This recipe is a favorite variation of regular chicken soup. The hot spices enhance the healing and comforting aspects of chicken soup. And the exotic taste is just right for a special meal. The two vegetables—the corn and avocado—make this a balanced meal.

Sweet Red Pepper and Crab Bisque

Yield: 6 servings	Serving size: ¾ cup	Prep time: 25 minutes	Cook time: 20 minutes
Each serving has:			
2 g carbohydrate	1 g fiber	16 g protein	

2 TB. butter

1 cup onion, chopped

1 cup celery, chopped

1 cup red bell pepper, chopped

1¼ tsp. seafood spice blend

3 cups fish stock or bottled clam juice

½ cup half-and-half

1 lb. fresh lump crabmeat

¼ tsp. cayenne

Salt and freshly ground black pepper to taste

1. Melt butter in a heavy, medium saucepan over low heat. Add onion, celery, red pepper, seafood spice blend, and fish stock. Cook, covered, for 10 minutes, stirring occasionally.

2. Add half-and-half. Bring to a simmer. Stir in crabmeat. Season with cayenne, salt, and pepper. Cover and turn off the heat. Let stand for 2 minutes. Ladle into soup bowls.

White Chili

Yield:	Serving size:	Prep time:	Cook time:
10 servings	1 cup	10 minutes plus 24 hours soaking time	6 hours

Each serving has:			
18 g carbohydrate	9 g fiber	29 g protein	

1 cup dry white northern beans	1 TB. ground cumin
7 cups chicken broth	$\frac{1}{2}$ tsp. ground cloves
2 cloves garlic, minced	1 (7-oz.) can green chilies, diced
1 large white onion, chopped	5 cups cooked chicken breast, diced
1 TB. ground white pepper	1 TB. jalapeño pepper, diced (optional)
1 tsp. salt	
1 TB. dried oregano	

1. Soak beans in water to cover for up to 24 hours; drain.

2. In a slow cooker or a large kettle, combine beans, $5\frac{1}{4}$ cups chicken broth, garlic, onion, white pepper, salt, oregano, cumin, and cloves. Simmer, covered, for at least 5 hours in slow cooker and $2\frac{1}{2}$ hours on stove until beans are tender, stirring occasionally.

3. Stir in green chilies, diced chicken, and remaining $1\frac{3}{4}$ cups chicken broth. For a hotter taste, add jalapeño (if using). Cover and simmer for 1 hour.

4. Spoon chili into soup bowls and serve.

RECIPE FOR SUCCESS

Beans are great for fiber and, combined with the chicken, make this a hearty dish. The south-of-the-border spices make this hot. To cool the temperature, omit the jalapeño pepper. Add avocado salad or guacamole on lettuce to make this a balanced meal.

Clam Chowder with Mushrooms

Yield:	Serving size:	Prep time:	Cook time:
6 servings	¾ cup	20 minutes	10 minutes

Each serving has:		
4 g carbohydrate	1 g fiber	16 g protein

2 TB. green onions, chopped

1 clove garlic, minced

4 TB. butter (½ stick)

1 lb. white mushrooms, sliced

2 TB. fresh parsley, chopped

2 TB. flour

2 (6.5-oz.) cans chopped clams with juice

2 cups water

Salt and pepper to taste

⅛ tsp. nutmeg

1½ cups heavy cream

1. Sauté green onions and garlic in butter. Add mushrooms and parsley, and cook 3 to 5 minutes longer until mushrooms are cooked throughout. Sprinkle with flour and stir. Add clams with juice, water, salt, pepper, and nutmeg. Bring to a boil, and simmer for 5 minutes. Add cream and reheat but don't boil.

2. Spoon chowder into soup bowls and serve.

RECIPE FOR SUCCESS

Try this clam chowder—it's filling, it's rich, it's creamy, and the mushrooms blended with the clams are fabulous.

Chicken Soup with Paprika

Yield:	Serving size:	Prep time:	Cook time:
6 servings	1 cup	20 minutes plus 30 minutes after cooking	1½ hours

Each serving has:		
2 g carbohydrate	1 g fiber	24 g protein

1 chicken breast	2 tsp. paprika
2 carrots, cut into 1-in. slices	½ tsp. thyme
2 leeks, trimmed and washed	1 bay leaf
1 tsp. salt	2 tsp. butter
Freshly ground black pepper to taste	3 large eggs, beaten
	2 TB. fresh parsley, chopped

1. To a soup kettle with 3 quarts water, add chicken, carrots, leeks, salt, pepper, paprika, thyme, and bay leaf. Bring water to a boil, and skim off any matter that rises to the top. Lower heat and simmer for 1½ hours. Remove bay leaf.

2. Remove chicken and let cool. Remove skin and de-bone chicken. Cut chicken into bite-size pieces.

3. Melt butter in a large skillet, and pour in eggs to make a very thin omelet. Cool and cut into shreds.

4. Add chicken, omelet shreds, and parsley to bouillon. Heat before serving.

RECIPE FOR SUCCESS

This is just the type of soup to use for a cold day, a head cold, and a heartwarming meal. The omelet shreds take the place of noodles. The soup tastes even better reheated. Serve with green beans, a salad, and a brownie or cookie for dessert.

Sweet-and-Sour Stew

Yield:	Serving size:	Prep time:	Cook time:
6 servings	¾ cup	25 minutes plus marinating overnight	1 hour, 15 minutes

Each serving has:		
10 g carbohydrate	2 g fiber	30 g protein

1½ lb. beef or pork, cut into cubes	2½ cups water
½ cup soy sauce	2 TB. vinegar
1 clove garlic, minced	1 tsp. molasses
4 TB. butter	½ cup pineapple chunks, water-packed, drained
1 green bell pepper, cut in strips	
2 medium onions, sliced	4 tomatoes, cut into wedges

1. Put meat into a resealable bag. Add soy sauce and garlic. Marinate overnight in the refrigerator.

2. Preheat the oven to 350°F.

3. Remove meat from marinade and discard marinade.

4. Sauté meat in 3 tablespoons butter until browned. Put into a large casserole. Sauté green pepper and onions in remaining 1 tablespoon butter. Add to the casserole. Combine water, vinegar, and molasses, stirring to blend. Pour over meat. Top with pineapple chunks and tomatoes.

5. Cover and bake for 1 hour and 15 minutes or until meat is tender.

RECIPE FOR SUCCESS

Here we have a taste of Asia—the sweet-and-sour taste—in a one-pot meal. Be sure to use water-packed pineapple. If you use juice-packed, the carb count increases by 7 grams.

Basic Cream Soup

Yield:	Serving size:	Prep time:	Cook time:
4 servings	½ cup	5 minutes	15 minutes

Each serving has:		
6 g carbohydrate	1 g fiber	4 g protein

1 cup heavy cream

1 TB. cornstarch

½ tsp. ground white pepper

½ tsp. cayenne

¼ tsp. salt

½ cup onion, minced or 3 TB. onion flakes

1 lb. white mushrooms, chopped, or 1 (8-oz.) can

1 TB. butter

1. In a cup, mix ¼ cup cream with cornstarch until smooth paste is formed. Over low heat, combine remaining ¾ cup cream, cornstarch mixture, white pepper, cayenne, salt, and onion. Stir constantly until mixture thickens, about 8 to 10 minutes. Remove from heat, and strain out onions through a mesh strainer and discard onions.

2. Sauté mushrooms in butter until softened; add strained soup, and stir over medium-low heat about 5 minutes or until thoroughly cooked.

RECIPE FOR SUCCESS

This is a wonderful fresh substitute for canned cream soups in any recipe. Substitute celery, cooked chicken, or other seasonings of choice for the mushrooms.

Beef–Vegetable Burgundy Stew

Yield:	Serving size:	Prep time:	Cook time:
6 servings	1 cup	10 minutes	2 hours

Each serving has:			
8 g carbohydrate	4 g fiber	29 g protein	

1 TB. butter

1½ lb. lean stew meat, cut into 1-in. pieces

1 tsp. thyme

1 tsp. freshly ground black pepper

1½ cups beef broth

¼ cup Burgundy wine

1 TB. garlic, minced

1½ cups carrots, sliced

1 cup pearl onions or 2 onions, quartered

1 (10-oz.) pkg. frozen English peas or soybeans

1. Melt butter in a Dutch oven, and brown beef cubes. Season with thyme and pepper. Stir in broth, wine, and garlic. Bring to a boil, reduce heat, cover, and simmer 1½ hours.

2. Add carrots, onions, and peas; simmer, covered, 30 minutes or until vegetables are tender.

RECIPE FOR SUCCESS

Let this hearty soup meant for cold wintry nights simmer while you begin your meal with Caesar Salad (see recipe in Chapter 20).

Cajun Black Bean Soup

Yield:	Serving size:	Prep time:	Cook time:
6 servings	1 cup	30 minutes	1 hour
Each serving has:			
10 g carbohydrate	3 g fiber	6 g protein	

2 cups cooked black beans, cooking liquid reserved

2 TB. butter

2 medium onions, chopped

1½ quarts (6 cups) beef or chicken broth

1 lemon, thinly sliced and seeds removed

1 TB. garlic powder

2 tsp. Cajun Spice Mix (see Chapter 12)

½ cup dry sherry

Salt to taste

Hot sauce to taste

2 large hard-boiled eggs, peeled and chopped

1. Mash 1 cup beans through a sieve; save remaining cup and set aside.

2. In a Dutch oven or heavy stew pot, melt butter and sauté onions. Add broth, mashed beans, and 2 cups reserved liquid from beans or enough water to make 2 quarts liquid for soup; stir well.

3. Add sliced lemon, garlic powder, Cajun Spice Mix, sherry, salt, and hot sauce. Simmer, covered, 1 hour.

4. Serve in soup bowls topped with chopped egg.

RECIPE FOR SUCCESS

One cup may not be enough of this Cajun delight! This soup makes a wonderful appetizer served in demitasse cups, as it is warm and inviting; just a taste won't fill up your guests before dinner but will make them beg for your recipe. It freezes well, so make a large amount to have on hand for those winter afternoons.

Catfish Stew

Yield:	Serving size:	Prep time:	Cook time:
6 servings	1 cup	10 minutes	40 minutes

Each serving has:			
8 g carbohydrate	2 g fiber	35 g protein	

2 lb. catfish nuggets (or cut fish fillets into bite-size nuggets)

Salt and pepper to taste

2 TB. butter

3 large onions, sliced

6 cloves garlic, minced (1 TB.)

2 drops hot sauce (optional)

1 (8-oz.) can tomato sauce

1 cup water

2 TB. Worcestershire sauce

1. Season fish with salt and pepper to taste and set aside.

2. Melt butter in a Dutch oven or stew pot, and sauté onions and garlic until soft. Stir in hot sauce (if using). Place fish nuggets on top of vegetables. In a small bowl, combine tomato sauce, water, and Worcestershire sauce. Pour mixture on top of fish, and simmer until fish flakes easily, about 30 minutes. Do not stir, as this will break up fish.

RECIPE FOR SUCCESS

This recipe is better if it's made early enough to allow the seasonings to be absorbed. You may add a bit more water, if desired, more juice, or serve over Vegetable Pasta (see recipe in Chapter 22) as a sauce. Add your favorite seasoning vegetables such as bell pepper, celery, mushrooms, etc. A salad and a luscious dessert completes this fish lover's meal.

Lentil Soup

Yield:	Serving size:	Prep time:	Cook time:
8 servings	¾ cup	10 minutes	1 hour cooking time for lentils

Each serving has:		
10 g carbohydrate	8 g fiber	7 g protein

1 cup dried lentils	1 TB. olive oil
4½ cups water	2 cloves garlic, minced
1 tsp. beef bouillon	½ tsp. dried oregano
1 onion, chopped	½ cup tomato sauce
2 carrots, chopped	2 TB. Worcestershire sauce
1 stalk celery, thinly sliced	

1. Place lentils in medium saucepan with 4½ cups water and bouillon. Bring to a boil, stirring to dissolve bouillon. Reduce heat and simmer for 1 hour until lentils are tender.

2. In a skillet, sauté onion, carrots, celery, garlic, and oregano in oil until tender. Stir in tomato sauce and Worcestershire sauce. Add mixture to lentil soup. Stir and serve.

RECIPE FOR SUCCESS

This hearty soup warms you on a chilly day and gives you energy to burn. Because it is low in complete protein, serve it as a side dish with meat, cheese, or pâté. Include a vegetable or salad, and you have a balanced meal.

Red Bean and Ham Soup

Yield:	Serving size:	Prep time:	Cook time:
8 servings	¾ cup	10 minutes	10 hours

Each serving has:		
17 g carbohydrate	6 g fiber	16 g protein

1 lb. ham, cooked and diced

3 cups cooked red beans

1 large red onion, chopped

1 (16-oz.) can tomatoes, diced

1 cup tomato sauce

1 TB. soy sauce

1 tsp. brown sugar

1 tsp. cayenne

½ tsp. dried basil

1. Place ham, red beans, red onion, tomatoes, tomato sauce, soy sauce, brown sugar, cayenne, and basil into a slow cooker; cook on low 8 to 10 hours. Add water as needed.

2. Spoon soup into soup bowls and serve.

RECIPE FOR SUCCESS

If you have a ham bone, add it to the pot for more delicious flavor. Add additional vegetables as you desire, and just calculate additional carbohydrates. This recipe makes a great base for a mixed vegetable soup for a cold winter day. Substitute leftover Thanksgiving turkey and the carcass for a wonderful heart- and tummy-warming November meal.

Rich Cheesy Soup

Yield:	Serving size:	Prep time:	Cook time:
6 servings	1 cup	10 minutes	30 minutes

Each serving has:		
9 g carbohydrate	1 g fiber	9 g protein

¼ cup butter

½ cup onion, minced

½ cup celery, diced

½ cup carrots, diced

¼ cup flour

3 cups chicken broth

3 cups heavy cream

1 cup cheddar cheese, shredded

½ tsp. ground white pepper

½ tsp. cayenne

2 TB. chives or green onions, finely chopped

1. In a stock pot, melt butter and sauté onion, celery, and carrots over low heat. Add flour slowly, stirring while cooking until thickened.

2. Add chicken broth. Pour in cream, and stir until smooth and bubbly. Add cheese, white pepper, and cayenne; stir until all cheese is melted and soup is smooth.

3. Sprinkle with chives when serving.

RECIPE FOR SUCCESS

This soup makes a wonderful accompaniment to a salad or served as a delightful sauce over steamed vegetables. Add or substitute additional cheeses as desired; Swiss cheese gives it a totally new flavor.

Basic Gumbo and Variations

Yield:	Serving size:	Prep time:	Cook time:
10 servings	1½ cups	1 hour plus cooking time for meat	2 hours

Each serving has:			
13 g carbohydrate	1 g fiber	24 g protein	

2 TB. butter

3 stalks celery, chopped

1 cup onion, finely chopped

3 garlic cloves, minced

3 qt. chicken broth

¼ cup flour

1 TB. Worcestershire sauce

½ cup fresh parsley, chopped or ¼ cup dried

½ tsp. cayenne

Salt and freshly ground black pepper to taste

1 tsp. Cajun Spice Mix (optional; see Blackened Fish recipe in Chapter 12)

6 cups cooked poultry or other meat choice (if using seafood it will cook in gumbo)

5 stalks green onions, chopped

Filé powder (optional)

1. Heat butter in a skillet, and sauté celery, onion, and garlic. Slowly stir in flour. Bring broth to boiling, pour slowly into the skillet mixture, stirring until thick and smooth; add sautéed vegetables, Worcestershire sauce, parsley, cayenne, salt, pepper, and Cajun Spice Mix (if using).

2. Add meat and simmer 2 hours for flavors to blend well. Add additional broth or water, if needed. If using seafood, add seafood for the last 30 minutes of cooking time. Add green onions the last 10 minutes of cooking. Serve with filé powder (if using).

3. Flavor is best if made at least 1 day in advance. Freezes well.

DEFINITION

Filé powder is ground sassafras root and is used in Southern-style cooking. It can be found in both grocery stores and specialty food stores.

Cajuns take their gumbo seriously! There are as many varieties of gumbo as there are people who eat it. Okra is said by some to be the main ingredient; others won't touch a gumbo if it has okra. Many use okra as the thickening agent. The basic recipe here omitted okra, but feel free to add 1 cup fresh or frozen okra if desired. The meat or seafood can be anything you want. You can use varieties of seafood such as shrimp, crawfish, crab (both flaked and in the shell), and oysters. Use wild game such as duck or squirrel as well as link sausage, rabbit, or chicken. Mix and match whatever you want. Just have fun and enjoy!

Shrimp Dinner Boil

Yield:	Serving size:	Prep time:	Cook time:
6 servings	12 large shrimp plus $\frac{1}{2}$ ear corn and $\frac{1}{2}$ onion	20 minutes	30 minutes

Each serving has:		
12 g carbohydrate	3 g fiber	18 g protein

$1\frac{1}{2}$ gallons water

1 lemon, cut into wedges

2 to 3 TB. crab boil or other seafood seasoning

$\frac{1}{4}$ cup salt

1 TB. freshly ground black pepper

6 dozen large shrimp (22–30 per lb.) still in shell

3 large ears corn, cut in half or use 6 small frozen ears of corn

3 medium onions, cut in half

1. In a large stock pot, bring water to a boil. Add lemon, crab boil, salt, and pepper.

2. Boil for 10 minutes. Add shrimp, corn, and onions, and bring back to boil. Boil 5 minutes; remove from heat and allow to stand covered 10 to 15 minutes. Pour into a large colander, or carefully spoon out vegetables and then drain shrimp.

3. Arrange vegetable and shrimp on a platter and serve.

RECIPE FOR SUCCESS

This can be considered a modified Louisiana Crawfish boil … only much easier and cooked indoors. Serve with ketchup seasoned with hot sauce.

Southern Chili

Yield:	Serving size:	Prep time:	Cook time:
6 servings	1 cup	20 minutes	2 hours

Each serving has:			
18 g carbohydrate	5 g fiber	31 g protein	

1 lb. ground beef

1 large onion, chopped

1 green pepper, chopped

1 (14.5-oz.) can tomatoes with jalapeños or chilies

1 (8-oz.) can tomato sauce

1 (14.5-oz.) can kidney beans, do not drain

2 tsp. chili powder

1 tsp. Cajun Spice Mix as in the recipe, Blackened Fish in Chapter 12

1 bay leaf

1 cup cheddar cheese, shredded, for garnish

1 cup sour cream, for garnish

3 green onions, chopped, for garnish

1. Brown beef and drain well; return to the skillet. In the same skillet, sauté onion and bell pepper until tender.

2. Add tomatoes, tomato sauce, kidney beans, chili powder, Cajun Spice Mix, and bay leaf; simmer 2 hours or pour into a slow cooker and heat on low 5 hours.

3. Remove bay leaf before serving. Garnish with shredded cheddar cheese, sour cream, and chopped green onions.

RECIPE FOR SUCCESS

Omit the beans if you wish and adjust the seasonings to your preference for hot or mild flavors. If you like a more tomato flavor, add 1 small can tomato paste and 1 can diced tomatoes.

Spicy Seafood Stew

Yield:	Serving size:	Prep time:	Cook time:
10 servings	1 cup	45 minutes	45 minutes (includes standing time)

Each serving has:		
4 g carbohydrate	2 g fiber	21 g protein

¼ cup butter

2 cups onion, chopped

½ cup celery, chopped

1 cup green bell pepper, chopped

2 TB. garlic, minced

4 cups chicken broth

1 (28-oz.) can stewed tomatoes, any seasoning

1 tsp. dill weed

1 tsp. freshly ground black pepper

½ tsp. cayenne

1½ lb. shrimp (45 large), peeled and deveined

2 dozen fresh or frozen crab fingers

1 (10-oz.) container oysters

Dash hot sauce (optional)

1. Melt butter in a Dutch oven or large skillet, and sauté onion, celery, bell pepper, and garlic until tender. Add broth, tomatoes, dill weed, black pepper, and cayenne. Simmer, uncovered, 20 minutes.

2. Add shrimp, crab fingers, and oysters. Add water or broth if additional juice is desired; cover and simmer 10 minutes. Stir in hot sauce (if using). Remove from heat and allow to stand covered 10 minutes before serving.

The Least You Need to Know

- Soups and stews warm the heart and the body for cold- and damp-weather meals.
- Scientists have actually proven that chicken soup is good at relieving cold and flu symptoms.
- Low-carb soups and stews provide a complete balanced meal and go well with warm fruit side dishes.
- Soups and stews are great for all meals—dinner, lunch, or breakfast.

Egg and Cheese Main Dishes

In This Chapter

- Keeping eggs and cheese on hand
- Recognizing good-for-you nutrition
- Making delicious meals with eggs and cheese

When you read the term "egg and cheese" dishes, please don't think "macaroni and cheese." Instead, expect even better. Yes, if you love the taste of eggy-cheesy food, you'll love the recipes in this chapter.

Egg and cheese dishes are great for any meal. Most of these recipes were created as dinner fare, but serve them whenever you want a rich, creamy taste and texture. For instance, an omelet, normally thought of as breakfast food, makes a hearty supper when filled with meat, cheese, or vegetables. (We have recipes for omelets in Chapter 5.)

Combinations of eggs and cheese yield different kinds of low-carb meals. Take a break from eating meat and vary your cuisine.

The Care of Eggs

Unless otherwise specified, these recipes call for whole eggs. Whole eggs work best. You could use egg substitutes or only egg whites, but we don't recommend it. The carbohydrate counts will be different, and you will lose some nutritional value.

Eggs will keep in the refrigerator for several weeks without going stale. But they are best when eaten within a week of purchase.

Grating Cheese

Want to save a few minutes of your busy life? Purchase pregrated cheese. If for some reason it's not available already grated or you got a great deal on a block of cheese, you'll need to grate it using one of these two methods:

- **With a hand grater.** This takes some elbow grease. Use a hand grater that can be draped over a bowl so the cheese falls inside neatly. One advantage of a hand grater is that you actually burn calories as you cook.

- **With a food processor.** Use the grating attachment and feed the cheese down the feeder tube while applying pressure with the pusher. It's quick and easy.

The Good Stuff in Eggs and Cheese

Eggs and cheese are both usually included under dairy products (although we suspect the chickens who laid the eggs would disagree). Both eggs and cheese offer good nutritional value in terms of protein and carbs. A cooked large egg has more than 6 grams complete protein and less than 1 gram carbohydrates.

The nutritional value of cheese varies based on the kind of cheese. One-quarter cup grated Parmesan contains 9 grams complete protein and 1 gram carbohydrate. The same amount of cheddar cheese has 6 grams complete protein and 1 gram carbohydrate.

Eggs and cheese are great for cooking because they blend with virtually every vegetable and fruit, spice and herb. Plus, eggs offer a soothing taste of their own, which can be spiced up with just the distinctive flavor of the added cheese.

Once upon a time, health experts thought that consuming eggs directly contributed to heart disease. Now they know better. Scientific studies show that consuming egg yolks doesn't appreciably elevate blood cholesterol levels. The lecithin found naturally in eggs may actually help the body clear out cholesterol. The real health concern isn't the cholesterol contained in the food you consume; it's the cholesterol level in your blood. Get that checked by your physician.

So there you have it. Not only are eggs not bad, they actually are good for you. So enjoy.

Whether you are eating low-carb for health reasons, heart reasons, or weight reasons, eggs and cheese combinations make excellent main dishes. Make a complete, balanced meal by adding vegetable and/or fruit side dishes to these recipes. Keep it light, as the dishes tend to be quite rich all by themselves. So think fresh salads, crudités, and fresh fruit platters.

Luncheon Egg Ring

Yield:	Serving size:	Prep time:	Cook time:
8 servings	$\frac{1}{8}$ ring	30 minutes	45 minutes
Each serving has:			
7 g carbohydrate	0 g fiber	35 g protein	

8 large eggs	1$\frac{1}{2}$ cups whole milk
2 cups whole milk, scalded	$\frac{1}{2}$ lb. (8-oz.) pkg. white mushrooms, sliced
1$\frac{1}{2}$ tsp. salt	
1 tsp. *onion juice*	1 lb. cooked chicken or 1 lb. crab
1 pinch cayenne	2 tsp. lemon juice
$\frac{1}{2}$ tsp. vegetable oil	$\frac{1}{4}$ tsp. paprika
5 TB. butter	Salt and freshly ground black pepper to taste
2 TB. flour	

1. Preheat the oven to 300°F.

2. Beat eggs slightly. With a whisk, mix in scalded milk, salt, onion juice, and cayenne. Strain egg mixture through a cheese cloth or a fine strainer. Pour into a well-oiled, 8$\frac{1}{2}$-inch ring mold with a bottom. Set in a shallow roasting pan filled with $\frac{1}{2}$ inch hot water, and bake 45 minutes or until firm.

3. In a large saucepan, melt 3 tablespoons butter, and stir in flour with a whisk. When blended, add milk, stirring constantly, until smooth and thickened. Remove from heat.

4. In a heavy skillet, sauté mushrooms in remaining 2 tablespoons butter over medium-high heat for 3 to 5 minutes. Add to cream sauce with chicken. Add lemon juice, paprika, salt, and pepper to taste. Heat to simmer, but do not boil.

5. When egg ring is baked, carefully loosen from the mold with a knife, and invert on a warm platter. Fill center and surround with cream mixture.

6. Slice to serve.

DEFINITION

Onion juice is a liquid seasoning similar to garlic juice and is packaged in a bottle. It can be found in the condiment aisle of your grocery store.

Chile Relleno and Crab Casserole

Yield:	Serving size:	Prep time:	Cook time:
10 servings	½ chile	20 minutes	45 minutes
Each serving has:			
8 g carbohydrate	5 g fiber	32 g protein	

1 (7-oz.) can whole, mild green chilies

1 lb. Monterey Jack cheese, cut into ¼-in.-thick slices

5 large eggs

1 (6.5-oz.) can flaked crabmeat

1¼ cups whole milk

¼ cup flour

½ tsp. salt

Dash freshly ground black pepper

4 cups (1 lb.) mild cheddar cheese, grated

1. Preheat the oven to 350°F.

2. Slit chilies lengthwise on one side. Remove seeds and drain. Place cheese inside chilies. Place stuffed chilies in an ungreased 3-quart baking dish or a soufflé dish.

3. Mix eggs, crabmeat, milk, flour, salt, and pepper well; pour over chilies. Sprinkle top with grated cheddar cheese. Bake uncovered for 45 minutes.

HOT POTATO

Purchase fresh, large eggs for these recipes. Open the carton and make sure none of them are cracked before you put the eggs in your grocery cart. Be careful when loading them into the car. Even eggs in cartons can crack and ultimately leak. Yuck.

Asparagus Cheese Pie

Yield:	Serving size:	Prep time:	Cook time:
8 servings	⅛ pie	20 minutes	35 minutes

Each serving has:			
4 g carbohydrate	1 g fiber	20 g protein	

1 lb. asparagus, trimmed, 6 spears reserved for top, the rest cut into ½-in. pieces	1 tsp. freshly ground black pepper
5 large eggs	½ tsp. ground nutmeg
15 oz. ricotta cheese	3 green onions, chopped, including tops
1 tsp. salt	½ lb. bacon, crisply cooked and crumbled

1. Preheat the oven to 375°F.

2. To a large pan of boiling water, add asparagus pieces, and cook 3 minutes. Drain, dry, and set aside.

3. In a large bowl, combine eggs, ricotta, salt, pepper, and nutmeg. Whisk to blend, and carefully stir in green onions, crumbled bacon, and cooked asparagus.

4. Spoon into a greased pie pan, and arrange reserved asparagus spears on top. Bake until firm, about 35 minutes.

RECIPE FOR SUCCESS

This recipe puffs up beautifully. It's a bit crusty on the outside, but it's creamy inside. It's fancy enough for guests and simple enough for dinner with your family.

Lemon Cheese Pie

Yield:	Serving size:	Prep time:	Cook time:
12 servings	$\frac{1}{12}$ pie	20 minutes	30 minutes

Each serving has:			
18 g carbohydrate	0 g fiber	3 g protein	

1 cup sugar

$1\frac{1}{2}$ TB. cardamom

$\frac{1}{4}$ cup butter

1 (8-oz.) pkg. cream cheese, softened

$1\frac{1}{2}$ TB. lemon zest, finely grated

$\frac{1}{3}$ cup sour cream

3 large egg yolks

1. Preheat the oven to 350°F.

2. In a small bowl, combine $\frac{1}{2}$ cup sugar and cardamom. In a large bowl with electric or hand mixer, beat $\frac{1}{4}$ cup butter and remaining $\frac{1}{2}$ cup sugar until smooth. Add cream cheese and lemon zest, and beat until fluffy. Blend in sour cream and egg yolks.

3. Pour into a buttered pie pan or quiche baking dish. Bake until golden brown and crisp, about 30 minutes. Cool and slice.

TABLE TALK

To make a low-carb pie crust, try this: Process 1 cup either almonds or pecans in a food processor until they turn into a flour, which is actually very finely chopped nuts. Add 1 egg and $\frac{1}{3}$ cup butter. Process as for pie dough. Spread dough into bottom of pie dish, and bake at 400°F for 10 to 13 minutes or until lightly browned. Let cool and fill. You can re-bake this with filling.

Cheese Apple Bake

Yield:	Serving size:	Prep time:	Cook time:
6 servings	5 slices apple	25 minutes	50 minutes

Each serving has:		
14 g carbohydrate	3 g fiber	3 g protein

¼ tsp. butter

4 medium baking apples (such as Fuji, Golden Delicious, or Granny Smith), peeled, cored, and cut into eighths

½ cup water

2 tsp. fresh lemon juice

¼ tsp. ground cinnamon

⅛ tsp. salt

½ cup cheddar cheese, shredded

1. Preheat the oven to 350°F.

2. In a shallow lightly buttered dish, arrange apple slices. Sprinkle with water and lemon juice. In a small bowl, combine cinnamon and salt. Sprinkle over apples.

3. Bake for 45 minutes or until apples are tender. Uncover. Top with shredded cheese. Bake for 5 more minutes or until cheese melts.

RECIPE FOR SUCCESS

Here's an apple treat that's low carb. The cheddar cheese adds complete protein. If you like more of a natural taste, don't peel the apples. Your children will find these hard to pass up—adults will, too!

Smoked Salmon Cheesecake

Yield:	Serving size:	Prep time:	Cook time:
12 servings	1 slice	30 minutes	2 hours, 20 minutes

Each serving has:		
5 g carbohydrate	0 g fiber	14 g protein

4½ TB. butter

¼ cup dry breadcrumbs

¾ cup grated Gruyère cheese

½ tsp. dill weed

1 medium onion, chopped

1 (8-oz.) pkg. cream cheese, softened

4 large eggs

⅓ cup half-and-half

½ tsp. salt

½ lb. smoked salmon, coarsely chopped

1. Preheat the oven to 325°F.

2. Butter an 8- or 9-inch springform pan, using about 1½ tablespoons butter.

3. In a small bowl, combine breadcrumbs, ¼ cup Gruyère cheese, and dill. Sprinkle mixture in the prepared pan, turning and tapping to coat evenly.

4. In a heavy skillet over low heat, melt remaining 3 tablespoons butter. Add onion, cover, and cook until soft, about 10 minutes.

5. In a food processor, blend cream cheese. Add eggs, remaining ½ cup Gruyère cheese, half-and-half, and salt. Process until smooth. By hand, stir in cooked onion and most of salmon, reserving 2 tablespoons. Pour into the prepared pan. Top with remaining salmon.

6. Wrap bottom of springform pan with aluminum foil. Set the pan in a large roasting pan filled with enough water to come halfway up the sides of the springform pan. Bake 80 minutes. Turn the oven off, and cool cheesecake in the oven with the door slightly ajar.

7. Cool to room temperature before removing the sides of pan. Cut into 12 slices, and serve at room temperature.

RECIPE FOR SUCCESS

This cheesecake even has a cheese crust! The combination of Gruyère cheese and smoked salmon is unique. The recipe makes plenty, so invite a crowd. Eat any leftovers for breakfast and lunch.

Chorizo Omelet

Yield:	Serving size:	Prep time:	Cook time:
6 servings	1 wedge	25 minutes	5 minutes
Each serving has:			
4 g carbohydrate	1 g fiber	18 g protein	

10 oz. *chorizo* sausage

1 cup onion, finely chopped

1 clove garlic, minced

1 TB. butter

1 cup green bell peppers, chopped

1 (4-oz.) jar pimiento, chopped

9 large eggs

½ tsp. salt

¼ tsp. freshly ground black pepper

DEFINITION

Chorizo is sausage flavored with Mexican spices and herbs. It's spicy!

1. In a large skillet, crumble chorizo and sauté until lightly browned. Drain and discard drippings.

2. Remove chorizo, and in the same skillet, sauté onion and garlic in butter. Add green peppers and pimiento, and cook 1 minute more. Stir in sausage.

3. In a large bowl, beat eggs with salt and pepper. Pour eggs over vegetables and sausage in the large skillet. Cook on one side, gently lifting the edges of the omelet to let the runny part run to the edges to cook, and then flip over. To flip, place a large plate upside down over the skillet. Invert the omelet onto the plate. Then gently slide the omelet back into the skillet.

4. Cut each half into 3 wedges before serving.

Eggs with Spinach

Yield:	Serving size:	Prep time:	Cook time:
4 servings	¼ recipe, which includes 2 eggs	25 minutes	10 minutes

Each serving has:		
11 g carbohydrate	0 g fiber	16 g protein

3 TB. butter	½ tsp. celery seed
3 TB. flour	Salt and freshly ground black pepper to taste
2 cups milk	½ cup spinach, chopped and cooked
½ tsp. dried ginger	8 large hard-boiled eggs, sliced
½ tsp. dried rosemary	
½ tsp. dried thyme	

1. In a heavy saucepan, melt butter. Add flour all at once and mix well. Cook a few minutes over low heat until butter-flour mixture is pale gold. Stir in milk with a wire whisk, stirring until mixture thickens.

2. Season with ginger, rosemary, thyme, celery seed, salt, and pepper. Gently stir in spinach and eggs.

3. Spoon into a 9 × 9-inch serving dish or platter. Serve warm or chilled.

TABLE TALK

If you're going to make 1 hard-boiled egg, you may as well make a half dozen or more. Eat them for snacks or make the Pickled Eggs recipe in Chapter 18. It's convenient to have hard-boiled eggs around, but just remember to eat them within a couple days.

Spinach and Ricotta Pie

Yield:	Serving size:	Prep time:	Cook time:
8 servings	1 slice	25 minutes	50 minutes

Each serving has:		
4 g carbohydrate	1 g fiber	16 g protein

1 (10-oz.) pkg. chopped frozen
 spinach

2 TB. butter

4 oz. prosciutto

1 garlic clove, minced

3 large eggs

¾ cup Parmesan cheese, grated

1 (15-oz.) pkg. ricotta cheese

Salt to taste

1. Preheat the oven to 375°F.

2. Cook spinach in a steamer over boiling water until tender. Drain and squeeze dry. Heat butter in a small skillet over medium heat. Add prosciutto and cook for 3 minutes. Stir in garlic, and remove from heat.

3. Beat eggs until lightly lemon colored. Add Parmesan cheese, ricotta cheese, spinach, prosciutto, and salt, and mix lightly.

4. Pour into a greased soufflé dish. Bake for 50 minutes or until done. Cut into 8 portions to serve.

RECIPE FOR SUCCESS

This is good-for-you food—low carb, complete protein, and a Mediterranean flavor. Serve with a tossed salad with romaine or Bibb lettuce. Choose a fruit soufflé or lemon mousse for dessert.

Cheesy Baked Eggs

Yield:	Serving size:	Prep time:	Cook time:
6 servings	1 egg	10 minutes	15 minutes

Each serving has:		
3 g carbohydrate	0 g fiber	11 g protein

4 TB. butter

1 medium onion, finely chopped

Salt and cayenne to taste

1 cup cheddar cheese, grated

6 large eggs

½ cup heavy cream or chicken broth

1. Preheat the oven to 350°F.

2. Melt butter in a skillet, and sauté onion until tender. Butter 6 individual baking dishes, and layer onions on the bottom, topped with salt, cayenne, and ½ cup cheese. Gently break each egg (without breaking yolks) onto cheese. Cover with cream, and top with remaining ½ cup cheese.

3. Cover dishes with foil, and bake 15 minutes until yolks are set and whites are cooked.

RECIPE FOR SUCCESS

Add additional seasonings to taste such as basil, dill, and oregano, or add shredded vegetables layered on top of onions such as squash or carrots. Refrigerate leftovers and eat the next day.

Cold Egg Cream Salad

Yield:	Serving size:	Prep time:	Cook time:
6 servings	2 halves with sauce	20 minutes plus time to chill	None

Each serving has:		
4 g carbohydrate	0 g fiber	7 g protein

6 hard-boiled eggs	3 TB. onion, minced
2 large egg yolks, beaten	1/4 cup celery, minced
2 TB. vinegar	1/2 cup heavy cream, whipped
2 TB. butter	1/4 cup mayonnaise
1/4 tsp. salt	6 sprigs fresh parsley
1/2 tsp. ground black pepper	1 tsp. paprika

1. Peel boiled eggs, and cut in half. Place in a serving bowl and set aside. Beat together egg yolks and vinegar, and cook over low heat, stirring until thickened. Set aside.

2. In a separate bowl, cream butter, salt, pepper, onion, and celery. Stir in egg yolk mixture and cool to room temperature.

3. Fold in whipped cream and mayonnaise.

4. Pour dressing over eggs in the serving bowl; garnish with parsley and paprika. Refrigerate and serve cold.

RECIPE FOR SUCCESS

This dish is perfect for those lazy dog days of summer. It makes a nice cool dish for a weekend brunch.

Sausage Muffins

Yield:	Serving size:	Prep time:	Cook time:
12 servings	1 muffin	15 minutes	25 minutes
Each serving has:			
3 g carbohydrate	0 g fiber	22 g protein	

½ lb. pork sausage, bulk

12 large eggs

½ cup onion, chopped

¼ cup green bell pepper, chopped

½ tsp. freshly ground black pepper

½ tsp. salt

¼ tsp. garlic powder

½ cup sharp cheddar cheese, shredded

1. Preheat the oven to 350°F.

2. Brown sausage and drain. In a separate bowl, beat eggs; add onion, bell pepper, black pepper, salt, and garlic powder. Stir in sausage and cheese.

3. Spoon into 12 muffin cups. Bake 20 to 25 minutes. Test doneness by inserting a knife into center of muffin. Muffins are done when the knife comes out clean.

RECIPE FOR SUCCESS

With no flour, these muffins are very low carb. They make the perfect breakfast, or use them as an accompaniment to soup and salad for lunch. When made in the tiny muffin tins, they make the perfect appetizer or party food.

The Least You Need to Know

- You get complete protein and low-carb eating with egg and cheese main dishes.
- Egg and cheese combinations are so versatile they blend well with a wide variety of fruits and vegetables.
- Egg and cheese meals are often quick and easy to make.
- Keep eggs and cheese in your refrigerator just in case you need them for a delicious dinner.

Salads Make a Meal

In This Chapter

- Not your everyday boring salads
- Salads mean low carb and high fiber
- Only the freshest ingredients

"More salads?" you're thinking. "Please, no." If you've been trying to eat healthy and eat low carb, the thought of more salads seems downright depressing. We understand. After years of salads for lunch, we're tired of salads, too. There's only so much lettuce anyone needs to eat in his or her lifetime.

We promise this chapter is filled with pleasant surprises, including some delicious main dish salads. We want you to toss out what's boring and instead toss salad ingredients with the most fragrant and wonderful dressings imaginable. You'll use walnut oil, chilies, and cilantro. You'll add curry and steak, even fennel and salami. You'll load your salads with dried cranberries, pine nuts, and capers.

These are salads fit for a king and for you. They're totally scrumptious, very low carb, and almost—shall we say—exciting! So read on, get out the salad bowl, and have fun. Great eating awaits you.

Low-Carb Salads

Vegetable salads are naturally low carb. With the main dish salads in this chapter, you also get plenty of complete protein because we include protein-rich ingredients. The total carb count, though, is somewhat higher than meat-only meals. That's because all vegetables contain carbohydrates. However, of all the categories of carbohydrates—starches, sugars, fruits, and vegetables—vegetables have the lowest counts.

Here's more good news. The lettuces and vegetables in these salads add fiber to your diet. Some people think that one drawback of a low-carb diet is a lack of dietary fiber. This is not true. Vegetables and fruits, such as you find in these recipes, give you plenty of fiber. You can definitely eat low carb *and* high fiber, especially if you conscientiously eat 5 to 10 servings of vegetables and fruits each day.

HOT POTATO

Some farmers' markets offer home and locally grown produce. But some vendors are a bit sneaky and sell produce from other regions of the country as well as produce imported from other countries. Be sure to check out the product's origin before you purchase!

Salad Ingredients

For most of these recipes you use raw vegetables, so you want the highest quality you can get. Organically grown versions are often available if you prefer them. In any case, go for the freshest and ripest you can find.

- **Fresh greens.** Select the freshest and ripest lettuces and vegetables. If the selection at the grocery store doesn't look that great, ask one of the produce specialists to bring out the back stock. Chances are good it's fresh and crisp.

- **Home grown.** If you have a vegetable garden, you already know the delights of fresh-picked lettuce and tomatoes. Vegetables don't get any better than home grown, although we suspect the love and sweat that went into growing them makes them taste even more delicious.

- **Oils.** Use only expeller-pressed oils. If an oil has been processed in any other way, it has been heated. Heat destroys the taste and the nutritional value. Plus, heat-processed oils could add unhealthy trans-fatty acids to your otherwise healthy salad. Store all expeller-pressed oils, such as walnut and canola, except olive oil in your refrigerator. Otherwise they may get rancid and end up tasting terrible.

- **Lemon and lime juice.** Your best choice is fresh squeezed. The second best choice is bottled organic fresh-squeezed juice with no preservatives. Your worst choice is bottled juice with preservatives.

- **Vinegars.** Vinegars are a delectable world unto themselves. Your choices include red or white wine vinegars as well as balsamic vinegars. There are many balsamic vinegars and a wide range of flavored varieties—red raspberry, tarragon, orange—you name it. When you find a favorite, use it in these recipes wherever vinegar is called for. Balsamic vinegar has a small amount of added sugar which brings out the delectable flavor. Don't be concerned with this small amount of carbs—it's negligible.

Pleasurable Salads

Eat salads because they taste good. Forget that they are also good for you, as that kind of thinking can ruin a delicious meal. Deep down, your body actually hungers for lots of this kind of food, so regularly make it part of your eating.

If you have room left after eating your salad, enjoy a wonderful dessert or chocolate treat (see Chapters 24 and 25, respectively).

Hot Chicken Salad

Yield: 6 servings	Serving size: ¾ cup	Prep time: 10 minutes	Cook time: 20 minutes
Each serving has: 6 g carbohydrate	2 g fiber	20 g protein	

2 TB. butter	¼ cup water or chicken broth
2 cups celery, diced	Salt and freshly ground black pepper to taste
½ cup slivered almonds	
1 cup green onions, chopped	2 TB. lemon juice
¼ cup mayonnaise	2 cups cooked chicken, cut into small pieces
1 (8-oz.) pkg. cream cheese, softened	Paprika, for garnish

1. Preheat the oven to 400°F.

2. Melt butter in a skillet, and sauté celery, almonds, and green onions until soft.

3. In a bowl, combine mayonnaise and cream cheese. Add water, salt, pepper, and lemon juice, stirring well until smooth. Add chicken and sautéed celery, almonds, and onions. Pour into a buttered baking dish.

4. Sprinkle with paprika, and bake for 20 minutes.

RECIPE FOR SUCCESS

This recipe is delicious served hot or cold. Substitute walnuts for almonds, and you'll be eating additional healthy omega-3 fats.

Steak Salad

Yield:	Serving size:	Prep time:	Cook time:
6 servings	1 cup	20 minutes plus 2 to 3 hours marinating time	None

Each serving plain salad has:		
4 g carbohydrate	2 g fiber	23 g protein

3 cups cooked roast beef, cut in thin strips

2 tomatoes, cut in wedges

1 green bell pepper, cut in strips

1 cup celery, sliced

⅓ cup green onions, sliced

⅓ cup white mushrooms, sliced

4 cups mixed greens (such as Bibb, leaf, or romaine lettuce, or Savoy cabbage)

Salad dressing #1:

Each 3 tablespoon serving has:		
5 g carbohydrate	0 g fiber	0 g protein

½ cup teriyaki sauce

⅓ cup dry sherry

⅓ cup salad oil

3 TB. cider vinegar

½ tsp. ground ginger

Salad dressing #2:

Each 3 tablespoon serving has:

| 1 g carbohydrate | 0 g fiber | 0 g protein |

½ tsp. salt

¼ tsp. pepper

3 dashes Tabasco sauce

¼ tsp. Worcestershire sauce

2 tsp. lemon juice

¼ cup red wine vinegar

1½ cups walnut oil

2 TB. green peppercorns

1. In a large bowl, combine beef, tomatoes, bell pepper, celery, onions, and mushrooms.

2. In a screw-top jar, combine ingredients for salad dressing of your choice. Shake well. Pour over beef mixture. Toss to coat well. Cover and refrigerate 2 or 3 hours.

3. Drain, reserving salad dressing.

4. Place greens in a large salad bowl; top with marinated meat and vegetables. Use reserved dressing at the table if anyone wants more.

RECIPE FOR SUCCESS

Rare roast beef isn't used often in salads, but the meat takes well to highly flavored dressings such as the ones in this recipe.

Scallop Salad

Yield:	Serving size:	Prep time:	Cook time:
4 servings	¼ recipe	20 minutes	10 minutes
Each serving has:			
5 g carbohydrate	2 g fiber	6 g protein	

½ cup dry white wine

¼ lb. bay scallops

6 TB. olive oil

1 TB. red wine vinegar

1 TB. balsamic vinegar

1 TB. fresh lemon juice

1 TB. fresh parsley, minced

½ tsp. salt

½ tsp. freshly ground black pepper

1 clove garlic, minced

1 medium tomato, chopped

1 small cucumber, chopped

2 stalks celery, chopped

1 small head red leaf lettuce

1 head Bibb lettuce, torn into pieces

1. To make salad, in a small saucepan, bring wine to a slow boil. Add scallops and cook until no longer transparent; drain.

2. To make dressing, combine olive oil, red wine vinegar, balsamic vinegar, lemon juice, parsley, salt, pepper, and garlic in a lidded jar and shake well.

3. Pour ⅓ of dressing over scallops; chill.

4. In a separate bowl, marinate tomato, cucumber, and celery in another ⅓ dressing; chill.

5. To serve, line 4 plates with red leaf lettuce. Top with Bibb lettuce. Divide marinated vegetables among the 4 plates. Arrange scallops on vegetables, and drizzle with remaining ⅓ dressing.

RECIPE FOR SUCCESS

The fresh ocean taste of scallops gives this salad a vacation feeling. You can enjoy it even in the winter months.

Seafood with Curried Chutney Dressing

Yield:	Serving size:	Prep time:	Cook time:
8 servings	⅛ recipe	30 minutes	None

Each serving has (without dressing):		
14 g carbohydrate	3 g fiber	29 g protein

Each 3 tablespoon serving of dressing has:
10 g carbohydrate

2 TB. peach or mango chutney	4 green onions, chopped
1 cup mayonnaise	1 lb. lump crabmeat
2 TB. tarragon vinegar	1 lb. shrimp (large, about 33 count), cooked, peeled, and deveined
2 TB. vegetable oil	1 cup cashews, toasted
2 tsp. curry powder	1 cup coconut, toasted
¼ cup half-and-half	1 cup raisins
1 head lettuce, torn into pieces	
4 stalks celery, chopped	

1. To make dressing, combine chutney, mayonnaise, vinegar, oil, curry powder, and half-and-half. Mix well.

2. To make salad, combine lettuce with celery and green onions; toss well. Arrange crabmeat and shrimp on top of lettuce, and drizzle with dressing. Sprinkle cashews, coconut, and raisins to taste over salad.

RECIPE FOR SUCCESS

This mixture has all the best tastes of curry in one dish—the cashews, coconut, raisins, and chutney. It transports you—at least in your taste buds—to a more exotic locale.

TABLE TALK

To toast coconut in the oven, set temperature to 350°F. Spread coconut in a thin layer in a large shallow baking pan. Put pan in the oven and toast for about 10 minutes, stirring every couple minutes until just lightly browned. It's best to toast the cashews in a separate pan, as they take about 5 minutes longer to turn golden brown.

Pacific Seafood Salad

Yield:	Serving size:	Prep time:	Cook time:
6 servings	⅙ recipe	20 minutes plus 1 hour marinating time	None

Each serving has:			
2 g carbohydrate	7 g fiber	24 g protein	

¼ cup olive oil

3 TB. red wine vinegar

1 TB. fresh lemon juice

2 tsp. Dijon mustard

1 tsp. anchovy paste

¼ tsp. freshly ground black pepper

1 lb. cooked tiny shrimp (65 count per pound), bay scallops, or a combination of both

4 tsp. Parmesan cheese, freshly grated

3 medium avocados, peeled and halved

3 cups Monterey Jack cheese, shredded

1. In a large bowl, place seafood. Combine oil, vinegar, lemon juice, mustard, anchovy paste, and pepper in a lidded jar and shake well. Pour dressing over seafood, and add Parmesan cheese; mix well. Marinate for 1 hour.

2. Place 1 avocado half in each of 6 individual ramekins. Divide seafood evenly among avocados. Sprinkle with Monterey Jack cheese. Place ramekins under heated broiler until cheese melts. Serve immediately.

RECIPE FOR SUCCESS

Many favorite flavors combine here for a refreshing main course salad. You can omit the anchovy paste and add 1 teaspoon capers, if desired.

Halibut Salad with Carrots and Fennel

Yield:	Serving size:	Prep time:	Cook time:
6 servings	1 halibut fillet plus ⅙ carrot and fennel mixture	30 minutes plus 30 minutes marinating time	10 minutes

Each serving has:		
4 g carbohydrate	2 g fiber	23 g protein

6 (4-oz.) halibut fillets

2 TB. olive oil

3 TB. orange juice

1 TB. fresh ginger root, minced

1 TB. freshly ground black pepper

1 tsp. jalapeño pepper, minced and seeded

For carrot-fennel salad:

2 cups carrots, shredded

2 cups fennel bulb, shredded

½ cup red vinegar

¼ cup olive oil

For dressing:

2 TB. orange juice

1 tsp. orange zest

½ cup olive oil

2 tsp. Dijon mustard

2 tsp. red wine vinegar

Salt and freshly ground black pepper to taste

1. Marinate halibut fillets in olive oil, orange juice, ginger root, black pepper, and jalapeño for at least 30 minutes. Before cooking halibut, combine carrots, fennel, vinegar, and oil.

2. Make dressing by combining orange juice, orange zest, olive oil, mustard, vinegar, salt, and pepper in a screw-top lid jar. Shake to blend.

3. Grill halibut over medium-high heat for about 4 minutes per side. Baste with marinade.

4. Spoon carrot-fennel salad onto individual serving plates. Place halibut fillets on top of salad. Spoon about 1 tablespoon dressing over each serving of halibut.

 RECIPE FOR SUCCESS

This recipe is a whole meal in a salad. The combination of fennel and carrots is unusual and enhances the halibut.

Chicken Cole Slaw

Yield:	Serving size:	Prep time:	Cook time:
10 servings	$\frac{1}{10}$ recipe	30 minutes plus 24 hours chill time	5 minutes

Each serving has:		
13 g carbohydrate	3 g fiber	15 g protein

3 cups chicken, shredded

1 head cabbage, sliced into $\frac{3}{8}$-in. strips

2 carrots, grated

1 green bell pepper, sliced into $\frac{1}{4}$-in. strips

1 red bell pepper, sliced into $\frac{1}{4}$-in. strips

1 (8-oz.) can water chestnuts

$\frac{1}{2}$ cup almonds, slivered

$\frac{1}{3}$ cup olive oil

$\frac{3}{4}$ cup cider vinegar

1 tsp. celery seed

1 tsp. salt

$\frac{1}{2}$ tsp. freshly ground black pepper

1. In a large bowl, combine chicken, cabbage, carrots, green and red bell peppers, water chestnuts, and almonds.

2. In a saucepan, heat oil, vinegar, celery seed, salt, and pepper to boiling. Pour over salad, toss, and refrigerate for 24 hours.

RECIPE FOR SUCCESS

Who would have thought to put chicken into a vinaigrette coleslaw? The results are simply good eating.

Beef Salad with Capers

Yield:	Serving size:	Prep time:	Cook time:
8 servings	$\frac{1}{6}$ recipe	30 minutes plus 3 hours marinating time	None

Each serving has (without dressing):		
4 g carbohydrate	2 g fiber	30 g protein

Each 2 tablespoon serving of dressing has:		
3 g carbohydrate	0 g fiber	0 g protein

For dressing:

4 tsp. capers

4 TB. fresh lemon juice

$\frac{1}{2}$ cup red wine vinegar

4 tsp. Dijon mustard

1 cup olive oil

$\frac{1}{2}$ tsp. freshly ground black pepper

1 tsp. sugar

For salad:

$1\frac{1}{2}$ lb. rare roast beef, cut into 1-in. strips

$\frac{3}{4}$ lb. fresh string beans, trimmed, blanched, and sliced

$\frac{1}{2}$ lb. white mushrooms, sliced

3 medium tomatoes, cut into wedges

1 (14-oz.) can hearts of palm, cut into rings

1 bunch watercress (2-3 cups), washed and stems removed

1 head romaine lettuce, torn into bite-size pieces

1. Prepare dressing by combining capers, lemon juice, vinegar, mustard, oil, pepper, and sugar. Pour about $\frac{1}{2}$ over beef, and marinate in the refrigerator for at least 3 hours.

2. Remove from refrigerator and add beans, mushrooms, tomatoes, hearts of palm, and watercress. Add additional dressing as needed.

3. Place lettuce on individual serving plates. Top with meat mixture.

4. Save extra salad dressing for later use.

RECIPE FOR SUCCESS

This is a completely balanced meal all by itself. It feels as if you are eating a rainbow. And you are—a rainbow of vegetables.

Oriental Spinach Salad

Yield:	Serving size:	Prep time:	Cook time:
8 servings	$\frac{1}{8}$ recipe	25 minutes	None
Each serving has:			
16 g carbohydrate	1 g fiber	16 g protein	

1 cup walnut oil

$\frac{1}{2}$ cup red wine vinegar

1 TB. Worcestershire sauce

1 (10-oz.) pkg. fresh spinach

8 oz. fresh bean sprouts

1 (8-oz.) can water chestnuts

4 large hard-boiled eggs, sliced

$\frac{1}{4}$ cup cashews

8 strips bacon, crisply fried and crumbled

8 slices salami, crisply fried and crumbled

1. In a small jar with a lid, place walnut oil, vinegar, and Worcestershire sauce. Secure lid and shake well to make dressing.

2. Wash, dry, and remove stems from spinach, then tear into pieces. Add bean sprouts, water chestnuts, eggs, cashews, bacon, and salami. Toss with dressing.

RECIPE FOR SUCCESS

This recipe makes a light main-course salad. For convenience and easier cleanup, use the microwave to cook the bacon and salami.

Artichokes Stuffed with Shrimp

Yield:	Serving size:	Prep time:	Cook time:
4 servings	1 artichoke plus ¼ shrimp-mayonnaise mixture	25 minutes	1 hour

Each serving has:		
7 g carbohydrate	7 g fiber	13 g protein

4 large artichokes

1 TB. Dijon mustard

2 TB. lemon juice

¼ cup mayonnaise

½ tsp. tarragon

Salt and freshly ground black pepper to taste

1 (6-oz.) can baby shrimp (get the really small ones)

1. Steam artichokes over boiling water for 1 hour or until done. Cool completely. Carefully open out artichoke leaves, and with a spoon, scrape out inner inedible part just above artichoke heart.

2. In a small bowl, combine mustard, lemon juice, mayonnaise, tarragon, salt, and pepper. Drain shrimp and stir into mayonnaise mixture.

3. Spoon shrimp mixture into hollowed-out part of each artichoke.

RECIPE FOR SUCCESS

Use the artichoke leaves to scoop out the shrimp for eating. When you finish eating the leaves, enough dressing should remain to eat the heart. It takes time to eat this salad—a major advantage to slowing down stress and enjoying the meal.

Asian Smoked Turkey Slaw

Yield:	Serving size:	Prep time:	Cook time:
6 servings	1 cup	20 minutes plus chill time	5 minutes

Each serving has:		
15 g carbohydrate	3 g fiber	19 g protein

1 cup fresh or frozen pea pods

2 TB. brown sugar

¼ cup rice vinegar

3 TB. olive oil

1 TB. sesame oil

4 cups Chinese cabbage, shredded

1 cup carrot, shredded

½ small red onion, sliced

½ small red onion, chopped

1 cup frozen green peas

Salt and freshly ground black pepper to taste

1 lb. smoked turkey, cut into small cubes or thin strips

6 red lettuce leaves

1. Blanch pea pods in boiling water for 2 minutes. Drain and set aside. Combine brown sugar, rice vinegar, olive oil, and sesame oil in a saucepan over medium heat and simmer.

2. In a large bowl, combine cabbage, carrot, sliced onion, chopped onion, pea pods, peas, salt, and pepper. Pour hot dressing over all and toss well. Add turkey and toss; chill. Serve 1 scoop in each lettuce leaf.

RECIPE FOR SUCCESS

What a light refreshing meal this is with just the right touch of sweet and sour with crunch! Serve with Parmesan Snacks (see recipe in Chapter 17) and tossed fresh fruit salad for a light lunch.

Basil Turkey with Peppers

Yield:	Serving size:	Prep time:	Cook time:
6 servings	½ cup turkey with 1 cup spinach salad	20 minutes	5 minutes

Each serving has:		
10 g carbohydrate	3 g fiber	23 g protein

2 TB. olive oil

1 green bell pepper, cut into 1-in. pieces

1 red bell pepper, cut into 1-in. pieces

1 TB. garlic, minced

3 cups cooked turkey, cubed

¼ cup fresh basil, chopped or 1 tsp. dried

6 TB. macadamia nuts, coarsely chopped

¼ cup balsamic vinegar

6 cups raw baby spinach leaves

3 cups grape or cherry tomatoes, sliced in half

1. Heat olive oil in a skillet, and sauté green bell pepper, red bell pepper, and garlic until tender. Mix in turkey cubes, basil, nuts, and vinegar; stir and cook for 5 minutes over medium heat.

2. Serve ½ cup turkey mixture over baby spinach with ½ cup sliced grape tomatoes. Pour any remaining hot dressing over salad; if needed, sprinkle salad with additional balsamic vinegar and olive oil.

 RECIPE FOR SUCCESS

This is a different take on the traditional hot spinach salad. Substitute any seafood or meat for the turkey for a change of flavor.

Chicken and Fresh Fruit Salad

Yield:	Serving size:	Prep time:	Cook time:
8 servings	1 cup	20 minutes plus 30 minutes chill time	None

Each serving has:			
14 g carbohydrate	3 g fiber	25 g protein	

3 cups cooked, boneless, cubed chicken

2 cups watermelon or cantaloupe, cubed

3 cups pears or peaches, cubed

1 cup fresh white mushrooms, chopped

$\frac{1}{2}$ lb. blue cheese, crumbled

2 cups sour cream

8 large lettuce leaves, such as romaine or Bibb lettuce

8 sprigs fresh mint, for garnish

$\frac{1}{4}$ cup almonds, slivered, for garnish

1. Combine chicken, watermelon, pears, mushrooms, blue cheese, and sour cream. Toss gently and then chill.

2. Serve on lettuce leaf, and garnish with mint sprig and a sprinkle of slivered almonds.

RECIPE FOR SUCCESS

This recipe is a complete meal as is. Add a vegetable, if you prefer, or save room for a rich chocolate dessert such as Chocolate Soufflé or a Double Chocolate Brownie—now that's planning ahead! Just look for both recipes in Chapter 25.

Grilled Fish Salad

Yield:	Serving size:	Prep time:	Cook time:
6 servings	1 cup	15 minutes	15 minutes to grill fish

Each serving has:		
12 g carbohydrate	1 g fiber	32 g protein

6 (5-oz.) fish fillets, baked or grilled

1 cup fresh baby spinach leaves, torn into bite-size pieces

4 cups fresh red leaf or green leaf lettuce, torn into bite-size pieces

1 cup cabbage, shredded

½ cup white mushrooms, sliced

½ cup green onions, chopped

6 marinated artichoke hearts, cut in half

For Garlic Mayonnaise:

1 tsp. minced garlic (can be found in the condiment section of your grocery store)

¾ cup mayonnaise

1. Grill or bake fish as desired. Place fish on individual plates.

2. In a large bowl, toss together spinach leaves, lettuce, cabbage, mushrooms, green onions, and artichoke hearts. Serve salad on top of hot or cold fish.

3. Combine garlic powder and mayonnaise, and drizzle each salad with 2 tablespoons Garlic Mayonnaise, vinaigrette, or other dressing of choice.

RECIPE FOR SUCCESS

This salad is actually best made with leftover grilled or baked fish. So next time you decide to have fish, cook extra to have on hand for this dish! It is such a light meal that you have room for a cup of soup and any scrumptious dessert.

Layered Roast Salad

Yield:	Serving size:	Prep time:	Cook time:
6 servings	1 cup	30 minutes plus chill time	None

Each serving has (dressing included):		
9 g carbohydrate	3 g fiber	25 g protein

4 cups lettuce, shredded

2 cups cauliflower florets

1 cup carrots, shredded

½ cup celery, sliced

1 lb. cooked roast beef, cut into bite-size pieces

1 cup chunky salsa

½ cup green onions, chopped

2 cucumbers, chopped

1 cup Green Goddess Dressing (see recipe in Chapter 20)

Paprika

Fresh parsley sprigs

1. In a large salad bowl, layer lettuce, cauliflower, carrots, celery, roast beef, salsa, green onions, and cucumbers. Spread Green Goddess Dressing over top, and refrigerate at least 30 minutes or overnight.

2. Just before serving, sprinkle with paprika for color, and add a few parsley sprigs for garnish.

RECIPE FOR SUCCESS

Vary this basic recipe to suit your taste. Use chicken instead of beef or Ranch dressing instead of Green Goddess; use any vegetables you prefer. This makes a beautiful presentation layered and served in a deep glass bowl.

Roasted Vegetable-Fruit-Beef Salad

Yield:	Serving size:	Prep time:	Cook time:
8 servings	1 cup mixed greens with 1 cup topping	15 minutes	30 minutes

Each serving has:			
14 g carbohydrate	1 g fiber	26 g protein	

2 zucchini, cut into 1-in. slices	$\frac{1}{4}$ cup balsamic vinegar
2 large red bell peppers, cut into 1-in. strips	1 TB. garlic, minced
2 onions, cut into 1-in. pieces	1 tsp. dried rosemary
18 white mushrooms, quartered	1 tsp. freshly ground black pepper
12 cherry tomatoes	4 TB. olive oil, divided
12 $1\frac{1}{2}$-in. cubes cantaloupe	$1\frac{1}{2}$ lb. beef steak, cut into strips
12 grapes	6 cups mixed greens

1. Preheat the oven to 425°F.

2. Place zucchini, bell peppers, onions, mushrooms, tomatoes, cantaloupe, and grapes on a greased baking sheet. Mix together vinegar, garlic, rosemary, pepper, and 2 tablespoons olive oil. Drizzle dressing on vegetables and fruit, and roast in the oven for 30 minutes, stirring once.

3. Stir-fry beef strips in a skillet in remaining 2 tablespoons olive oil until done, about 10 minutes.

4. Arrange beef strips over mixed greens, and top with hot vegetables and fruit. If additional dressing is needed, sprinkle with olive oil and balsamic vinegar.

RECIPE FOR SUCCESS

Roasted fruit is an unusual treat for many; experiment with other fruits or even double up on veggies and omit fruit for a lower carb count.

Turkey-Apple Salad

Yield:	Serving size:	Prep time:	Cook time:
8 servings	¾ cup	15 minutes plus chill time	None

Each serving has:			
13 g carbohydrate	2 g fiber	26 g protein	

2 cups boneless turkey or chicken, diced and cooked

2 cups red or green apples, diced

½ cup walnuts, chopped or other nuts of choice

½ cup celery, chopped

½ cup mayonnaise

2 TB. brown sugar

3 TB. spicy brown mustard

Dash dried rosemary

Salt and freshly ground black pepper to taste

6 red lettuce leaves

1. Combine turkey, apples, walnuts, and celery; set aside.

2. In a small bowl, combine mayonnaise, brown sugar, mustard, rosemary, salt, and pepper.

3. Combine mayonnaise mixture with turkey mixture and chill. Serve 1 scoop of turkey salad on red lettuce leaf.

RECIPE FOR SUCCESS

What a refreshing summer lunch this is or the perfect take-along meal any time of the year! Serve with a cold fruit or vegetable soup for a completely satisfying meal.

The Least You Need to Know

- Main dish salads are a superb, delicious way to eat a balanced meal.
- Main dish salads are wonderfully varied, interesting, and delicious.
- Make salad dressings with olive oil and other expeller-pressed raw oils such as walnut oil.
- Salads are deeply satisfying when you can get beyond eating them only because they are good for you.

Side Dishes

Snacks and appetizers give you plenty of variety for in-between-meal munching and entertaining. From Parmesan crackers to a chocolate chip cheese appetizer, these low-carb treats satisfy your hunger and your taste buds.

Vegetables, fruits, and side salads rate a chapter each. You'll have an easy time eating enough fruits and vegetables with these low-carb recipes. Prepare them to accompany main dish entrées in Parts 3 and 4, and get set to love eating your veggies!

Appetizers

In This Chapter

- Eating before meals
- Recognizing low-carb appetizers
- Eating low carb at cocktail parties
- Making a meal of appetizers

Cocktail parties are one of the easiest places to eat low carb naturally—provided the host or hostess prepared traditional appetizers such as meatballs, water chestnuts wrapped in bacon, crudités, cheese cubes, chicken livers wrapped in bacon, shrimp cocktail, or deviled eggs.

The list of delicious low-carb tidbits goes on and on. You could make a whole meal of low-carb appetizers … and plenty of us have done just that! At a party you may want to forego the chips, but, happily, you usually can enjoy the dip by using a vegetable scooper. When you are hungry for appealing bites of low-carb foods, traditional appetizers such as vegetables, meats, fish, and cheese make for delightful eating.

Unfortunately, party givers often serve breads and starchy foods in place of low-carb fare at many of today's cocktail buffets. If you attend one of these parties, you'll need to carefully choose what you eat.

And remember, when it's your turn to throw a party, make sure your spread includes lots of low-carb yummies.

Bite-Size Low Carb

Virtually all traditional appetizers are low carb. You can usually expect to find meats, fish, cheese, or seafood, with or without vegetables and fruit. The recipes in this chapter are mostly high protein plus a couple vegetable offerings. Definitely, they are no starch and totally delicious.

On the menus of many restaurants, the appetizers look more appealing than the entrées. So go ahead and order one or two appetizers and a side salad for your meal. You'll find that you're totally satisfied. It's also a good approach to consider for your own meals and parties.

Beauty, the saying goes, lies in the eye of the beholder. This may explain why appetizers are so appealing. Presented well, appetizers look marvelously delicious. Fortunately, even the simplest appetizers can appear quite elegant. We know you have better things to do than spend unnecessary time in the kitchen, so these recipes use simple preparation techniques whenever possible.

TABLE TALK

Have you ever showed up hungry to a party only to discover that there isn't any low-carb food to eat? Picking the chunks of chicken out of the chicken salad definitely seems out of place and unappreciative. To prevent this scenario from happening again, take the hostess a gift of a low-carb appetizer. Make sure the one you prepare has plenty of complete protein. Cook enough for everyone to enjoy and for you to have your fair share … and maybe seconds.

History of Before-Meal Hunger

Very few people can actually wait to eat until dinnertime—at least not people we know. Only those mythological people we have never met can actually go from lunch until 7 or 8 P.M. in the evening without eating. If we have to wait 7 or 8 hours before eating again, when dinner is finally served, we don't eat, we inhale. This is not good. Rapidly consuming food often leads to overeating, indigestion, and weight gain.

Appetizers solve this problem. Traditionally, appetizers are served anywhere from $\frac{1}{2}$ to 1 hour or even 2 hours before dinner. The length of time often depends on how much alcohol people are willing to drink before they eat, but that's another matter entirely.

The appetizer is the traditional solution to the problem of acute "I'm-ready-to-eat-the-napkins" ravenous hunger. It contains enough food and nourishment to tide you over until dinner is served. The key is to eat a few appetizers but not too many, or dinner won't seem appealing.

As to the alcohol consumption at this pre-dinner time, you'll need to judge how much is fine, how much is enough, and how much is sloppy. Too much will obviously impair your ability to enjoy your food and perhaps to make discriminating food choices.

Parmesan Snacks

Yield:	Serving size:	Prep time:	Cook time:
8 servings	$\frac{1}{4}$ ounces cheese	5 minutes	10 minutes

Each serving has:			
1 g net carbohydrate	0 g fiber	8 g protein	

1½ cups Parmesan cheese,
    shredded

1. Preheat the oven to 400°F.

2. Spread cheese in a thin layer on a cookie sheet covered with a silicone baking sheet liner or parchment paper.

3. Bake for 10 to 12 minutes until cheese is lightly toasted and browned. Cool, break into pieces, and serve.

RECIPE FOR SUCCESS

Everyone likes these Parmesan snacks—they disappear really fast. If you should have any left over, crumble and sprinkle on salads and steamed vegetables.

Chocolate-Chip Cheese Ball

Yield:	Serving size:	Prep time:	Cook time:
20 servings	½ ball or or 2½ tablespoons	20 minutes plus 3 hours chill time	None

Each serving has:			
6 g carbohydrate	1 g fiber	2 g protein	

1 (8-oz.) pkg. cream cheese, softened

½ cup butter (no substitutes), softened

¼ tsp. vanilla extract

2 TB. confectioners' sugar

2 TB. brown sugar

¾ cup miniature semi-sweet chocolate chips

¾ cup pecans, finely chopped

1. In a mixing bowl, beat cream cheese, butter, and vanilla until fluffy. Gradually add confectioners' and brown sugars; beat just until combined. Stir in chocolate chips.

2. Cover and refrigerate for 2 hours. Place cream cheese mixture on a large piece of plastic wrap; shape into a ball.

3. Refrigerate ball for at least 1 hour. Just before serving, roll cheese ball in pecans.

Brie Stuffed with Sun-Dried Tomatoes and Basil

Yield:	Serving size:	Prep time:	Cook time:
6 servings	⅙ recipe	20 minutes	None

Each serving has:			
4 g carbohydrate	1 g fiber	8 g protein	

½ cup fresh basil, chopped

10 oil-packed, sun-dried tomatoes, drained (reserve oil)

2 garlic cloves, peeled

¼ tsp. freshly ground black pepper

1 tsp. fresh lemon juice

1 wedge Brie cheese (about ½ lb.), thoroughly chilled

1. In a food processor, combine basil, sun-dried tomatoes, garlic, pepper, and lemon juice. Process until paste forms. Add oil from sun-dried tomatoes or olive oil if texture is very dry. Mixture needs to be spreadable, but not runny.

2. Cut Brie in half horizontally. Spread bottom half with reserved sun-dried tomato mixture, and top with remaining half, pressing halves together firmly. Chill in the refrigerator and then bring to room temperature before serving.

RECIPE FOR SUCCESS

You can eat this delicious appetizer with a fork or spread on slices of jicama, celery root, and other vegetables. You may prepare this recipe 1 day in advance. Serve chilled or at room temperature.

Lobster with Mango

Yield:	Serving size:	Prep time:	Cook time:
6 servings	1/6 recipe, about 1/2 cup lobster plus 1/6 mango and sauce	20 minutes	None

Each serving has:		
12 g carbohydrate	1 g fiber	27 g protein

1 tsp. ginger root, minced	2 mangos, halved and pitted
4 TB. olive oil	1 1/2 cups cooked lobster meat
2 TB. lemon juice	4 sprigs fresh mint

1. Mix ginger root with olive oil and lemon juice and set aside.

2. Remove pulp from mangos, and cut into bite-size pieces. Divide among 4 small plates. Place lobster meat beside mango, and top with a sprig of mint.

3. Spoon ginger sauce on top of lobster and mango, and serve.

RECIPE FOR SUCCESS

Serve this simple, tasty, and exotic recipe as an appetizer or increase the serving size and serve as a main dish salad on a bed of Bibb lettuce. You can also substitute shrimp for the lobster.

Lobster Pâté

Yield:	Serving size:	Prep time:	Cook time:
10 servings	¼ cup	15 minutes plus several hours chill time	None

Each serving has:		
2 g carbohydrate	0 g fiber	17 g protein

1 (8-oz.) pkg. cream cheese, softened

¼ cup dry white wine

½ tsp. salt

⅛ tsp. fresh cilantro, chopped

1½ cups lobster meat, finely chopped

1. Beat cream cheese and wine with salt and cilantro until smooth. Stir in lobster. Cover and refrigerate several hours or more.

Smoked Salmon Spread

Yield:	Serving size:	Prep time:	Cook time:
6 servings	¼ cup	15 minutes plus 1 hour chill time	None

Each serving has:		
0 g carbohydrate	0 g fiber	4 g protein

4 oz. smoked salmon

2 dashes hot sauce

2 dashes Worcestershire sauce

Freshly ground black pepper to taste

½ cup whipping cream

1. In a food processor, process salmon, hot sauce, Worcestershire sauce, and pepper until smooth. Whip cream in a bowl until stiff peaks form. Fold in salmon mixture. Refrigerate for 1 hour or more.

2. Serve on individual plates on top of lettuce leaves, or serve as a dip with vegetable crudités, such as carrots, jicama, and celery.

HOT POTATO

The pâtés and spreads in this chapter are low carb. Be sure to follow our serving suggestions to keep them low carb. Don't eat them with regular crackers or breads, or the carb count will go up fast.

Avocado Margarita

Yield:	Serving size:	Prep time:	Cook time:
8 servings	⅛ recipe	20 minutes	None

Each serving has:			
1 g carbohydrate	4 g fiber	1 g protein	

1 TB. onion, minced

2 TB. fresh cilantro, chopped

Salt and freshly ground black pepper to taste

Juice 1 lime

2 medium avocados

1 medium tomato, chopped

1. In a small bowl, mix onion, cilantro, salt, pepper, and lime juice.

2. Cut open avocados, remove pits, and spoon out fruit into a bowl. With a spoon, cut any big chunks of avocado into smaller ones, but keep chunks quite large—1 inch square is fine. Add chopped tomato. Add onion mixture, and stir gently to blend.

3. Serve as a side dish to meat, seafood, and poultry dishes.

RECIPE FOR SUCCESS

The secret is in the lime juice and the big chunks of avocado. When my friend brought this Margarita to a potluck, it was gone before we could turn around for seconds. We loved it.

Spinach Cheese Squares

Yield:	Serving size:	Prep time:	Cook time:
20 servings	2 squares	15 minutes	35 minutes

Each serving has:			
4 g carbohydrate	0 g fiber	8 g protein	

½ cup butter (1 stick)	1 tsp. salt
3 eggs	1 tsp. baking powder
½ cup flour	1 lb. Monterey Jack cheese, grated
1 cup milk	4 cups fresh spinach, chopped

1. Preheat the oven to 350°F.

2. Melt butter in a 9 × 13-inch pan.

3. Beat eggs, adding flour, milk, salt, and baking powder. Add cheese and spinach to the bowl, mixing well.

4. Pour mixture into the pan, and bake 35 minutes. Cool before serving. Cut into squares.

Deviled Eggs

Yield:	Serving size:	Prep time:	Cook time:
6 servings	4 halves	25 minutes plus chill time	None

Each serving has:			
1 g carbohydrate	0 g fiber	13 g protein	

12 hard-boiled eggs	Salt and freshly ground black pepper to taste
Mayonnaise	¼ tsp. paprika

1. Peel and cut each egg in half lengthwise, and gently remove yolks, saving whites to refill.

2. Put all yolks in a bowl, and gently moisten with just enough mayonnaise so they hold together. Add salt and pepper to taste and paprika. Refrigerate until serving.

3. You can repack eggs with yolk mixture as is, or you can add more zest. See following variations.

Variations: These additions will have little effect on the carb count: dry mustard; cayenne; curry powder; caviar; minced ham, bacon, or beef; grated Parmesan or Roquefort cheese; chopped fresh cilantro, basil, rosemary, tarragon, or chopped ginger. These could slightly increase carb count: chutney, chopped black or green olives; capers; chopped dill pickles; or minced onion. You can combine them if you like.

RECIPE FOR SUCCESS

Deviled eggs contain terrific protein and work well as hostess gifts for parties or to take to potluck dinners. It seems everyone loves deviled eggs—they're usually gone within 10 minutes of setting out the serving tray.

TABLE TALK

Adding grated Parmesan cheese to any of the combinations—whether sweet or savory—enhances the flavor and will have guests asking for your "secret" ingredient.

Baked Avocado

Yield:	Serving size:	Prep time:	Cook time:
6 servings	½ avocado	20 minutes	10 minutes
Each serving has:			
5 g carbohydrate	7 g fiber	6 g protein	

3 large avocados

1 lemon

Salt to taste

3 hard-boiled eggs, peeled and chopped

¼ cup celery, finely chopped

¼ cup red bell pepper, finely chopped

2 TB. onion, finely chopped

½ tsp. cayenne

¼ cup mayonnaise

3 TB. pine nuts, almonds, or walnuts, chopped, for garnish

1. Preheat the oven to 400°F.

2. Cut avocados in half, leaving peel intact; remove pit. Cut lemon in half, and sprinkle each cut side of avocado with lemon juice to prevent browning; sprinkle with salt.

3. Combine eggs, celery, red bell pepper, onion, cayenne, and mayonnaise.

4. Fill each avocado half with scoop of egg mixture, and place on a baking pan. Bake 10 minutes. Sprinkle with nuts and serve.

RECIPE FOR SUCCESS

Cooked chicken or seafood may be added to mixture to fill avocados, if desired. For the main dish, make a larger batch with added protein and bake in a casserole dish without the avocado. To serve, place lettuce or cabbage leaf onto a plate, scoop cooked mixture onto the leaf, and top with sliced avocado.

Baked Swiss Onion Dip

Yield:	Serving size:	Prep time:	Cook time:
24 servings	¼ cup	15 minutes	30 minutes
Each serving has:			
5 g carbohydrate	1 g fiber	3 g protein	

3 sweet onions, chopped in large pieces

2 TB. butter

2 cups (8-oz.) pkg. shredded Swiss cheese

1 cup sour cream

1 cup mayonnaise

¼ cup white wine

½ tsp. cayenne

1 tsp. white pepper

1 tsp. garlic powder

1. Preheat the oven to 375°F.

2. In a large skillet over medium heat, sauté onions in butter until tender. Add cheese, sour cream, mayonnaise, wine, cayenne, white pepper, and garlic powder to the pan; stir well until blended.

3. Pour mixture into a baking dish, and bake 30 minutes. Let stand 10 minutes before serving.

Broccoli-Seafood Dip

Yield:	Serving size:	Prep time:	Cook time:
16 servings	¼ cup	15 minutes	15 minutes
Each serving has:			
3 g carbohydrate	1 g fiber	10 g protein	

2 TB. butter

½ cup onion, finely chopped

½ lb. white mushrooms, sliced

1 (10-oz.) pkg. frozen broccoli, chopped

1 tsp. Worcestershire sauce

8 oz. processed cheese block, chopped into small pieces

1 tsp. freshly ground black pepper

½ tsp. cayenne

1 lb. cooked crawfish tails, peeled shrimp, or crabmeat

1 cup sour cream

¼ cup water (optional)

1. Melt butter in a skillet, and sauté chopped onion and mushrooms until tender; add broccoli, Worcestershire sauce, cheese, black pepper, and cayenne, and stir until heated through. Stir in seafood and sour cream, and bring to simmer for 5 minutes. Serve with vegetable dippers.

Variations: Substitute cooked ground beef or shredded chicken for the seafood. As a main dish, serve over Vegetable Pasta (see recipe in Chapter 22).

Chicken Quesadillas

Yield:	Serving size:	Prep time:	Cook time:
6 servings	1 tortilla	20 minutes	20 minutes
Each serving has:			
10 g carbohydrate	3 g fiber	30 g protein	

2 TB. butter

1 red bell pepper, chopped

3 green onions, chopped

1 TB. garlic, minced

3 cups cooked chicken, shredded

$\frac{1}{2}$ cup fresh cilantro or parsley, finely chopped

6 low-carb tortillas

$\frac{2}{3}$ cup cheddar cheese, shredded

$\frac{2}{3}$ cup Monterey Jack cheese, shredded

$\frac{3}{4}$ cup sour cream

$\frac{3}{4}$ cup guacamole

1 cup salsa

1. Preheat the oven to 250°F.

2. Melt butter in a large skillet, and sauté bell pepper, onions, and garlic. Stir in chicken and cilantro and heat.

3. Place 2 tablespoons chicken mixture in center of each tortilla, top with $1\frac{1}{2}$ tablespoons each cheddar and Monterey Jack cheeses, and fold in half. Set aside until all tortillas are filled.

4. Heat a large skillet, or fire up the grill. Add 1 or 2 quesadillas, and cook over medium heat for 2 to 3 minutes. Flip and cook until cheese is completely melted, another minute or so.

5. Repeat with all tortillas, stacking them on a baking sheet and keeping them warm in the oven while cooking others.

6. To serve, place 1 quesadilla on a plate, cut into 4 wedges, and top each wedge with $\frac{1}{2}$ tablespoon each sour cream and guacamole. Pour $\frac{1}{4}$ cup salsa into individual ramekins for each plate to dip wedges.

RECIPE FOR SUCCESS

To lower your carb count by 7 grams per tortilla, pile up the ingredients on a plate, warm in microwave a few seconds to melt the cheese, and top with sour cream and guacamole … just as tasty! Another option is to fill a cabbage leaf instead of a tortilla and heat in the same manner to melt the cheese.

Eggplant Spread

Yield:	Serving size:	Prep time:	Cook time:
6 servings	$\frac{1}{2}$ cup	10 minutes	35 minutes
Each serving has:			
6 g carbohydrate	8 g fiber	3 g protein	

2 large eggplants

$1\frac{1}{4}$ cups fresh basil or 1 TB. dried

2 TB. garlic, minced

20 green olives, pitted

Salt and freshly ground black pepper to taste

1. Preheat the oven to 375°F.

2. Butter a baking pan, and cover with foil if desired. Cut eggplants in half lengthwise, and lay cut side down on the pan. Bake until eggplant is soft, about 35 minutes. Cool.

3. Scrape pulp out of eggplant shells. Blend in food processor with basil, garlic, olives, salt, and pepper. Let stand at room temperature before serving.

Hot Crab Dip

Yield:	Serving size:	Prep time:	Cook time:
6 servings	$\frac{1}{4}$ cup	10 minutes	25 minutes
Each serving has:			
2 g carbohydrate	< 1 g fiber	10 g protein	

1 (7-oz.) can crab or fresh lump crabmeat

1 (8-oz.) pkg. cream cheese, softened

$\frac{1}{2}$ tsp. horseradish

1 TB. sherry or cream

2 TB. onion, chopped

2 tsp. garlic, minced

1 tsp. ground white pepper

$\frac{1}{4}$ cup shredded cheese of choice

1. Preheat the oven to 375°F.

2. Blend crab, cream cheese, horseradish, sherry, onion, garlic, and white pepper, and pour into a greased baking dish.

3. Bake for 15 minutes, sprinkle with shredded cheese, and return to oven for 10 minutes or until cheese is melted and bubbly.

4. Serve with vegetable scoopers.

RECIPE FOR SUCCESS

Use this basic creamy dip to create your own unique dip. Add in whatever seasonings you prefer, such as dill weed or basil. Change the protein base to shredded chicken or chipped beef, etc. You can also add chopped artichoke hearts, asparagus, spinach, or broccoli. Top with nuts, or for a unique blend of flavors you might add golden raisins. Let your creative juices flow!

Marinated Crab Fingers

Yield:	Serving size:	Prep time:	Cook time:
6 servings	3 tablespoons	10 minutes plus overnight marinating time	None

Each serving has:		
0 g carbohydrate	0 g fiber	5 g protein

1 tsp. dried basil

1 tsp. dry mustard

1 TB. garlic, minced or 1 tsp. garlic powder

$\frac{1}{2}$ tsp. salt

$\frac{1}{2}$ tsp. freshly ground black pepper

$\frac{1}{2}$ tsp. cayenne

3 TB. balsamic vinegar

1 TB. lemon juice

1 TB. Worcestershire sauce

2 TB. white wine or white cranapple juice made without added sugars or sweeteners

2 TB. olive oil

1 lb. crab fingers or crab claws

1. In a medium bowl with a tight-fitting lid, combine basil, dry mustard, garlic, salt, pepper, cayenne, vinegar, lemon juice, Worcestershire sauce, wine, and oil; shake well. Add crab fingers, and gently shake to cover well. Marinate in the refrigerator overnight, turning over several times to coat fingers well.

2. Drain marinade before serving.

The marinade makes a delicious salad dressing. Serve crab fingers over red leaf lettuce as a salad. Sprinkle with parsley. This dressing also makes a wonderful dipping sauce for artichoke leaves.

Eat crab fingers just like you would artichoke leaves. Grab the claw by the pincher hook and bite, pulling off the meat with your teeth.

Mushroom "Caviar"

Yield:	Serving size:	Prep time:	Cook time:
6 servings	2 tablespoons	30 minutes plus chill time	None

Each serving has:		
3 g carbohydrate	1 g fiber	1 g protein

½ lb. white mushrooms, finely chopped

1 onion, finely chopped

2 TB. olive oil

Juice 1 lemon

Freshly ground black pepper to taste

1. In a skillet over low heat, sauté mushrooms and onion in oil until tender.

2. Add lemon juice and pepper, and simmer 15 to 20 minutes. Refrigerate and serve chilled.

Surprise your guests and serve this caviar at your next party. It is great served in Belgium endive leaves or small celery boats. Make plenty, as it goes fast. This mushroom caviar also makes a great topping on salads and vegetables or use as a garnish for cheese balls.

Olive Cheese Bites

Yield:	Serving size:	Prep time:	Cook time:
Approx. 50 bites	2 pieces	20 minutes plus freezing overnight	15 minutes

Each serving has:			
5 g carbohydrate	1 g fiber	4 g protein	

2½ cups cheddar cheese, grated
¾ cup butter (1½ sticks), softened
1¼ cups all-purpose flour
1 tsp. cayenne

1 tsp. paprika
100 small stuffed olives

1. These bites should be made at least 1 day in advance to allow for freezing.

2. On day of baking, preheat the oven to 400°F.

3. Blend cheese and butter; stir in flour, cayenne, and paprika, and mix well. Wrap 1 teaspoon cheese mixture around each olive; cover completely.

4. Best if frozen at this stage and baked when frozen. To freeze, place on sheet pans and freeze until firm; if desired, remove to freezer storage bags until ready to bake.

5. Place cheese bites on a baking sheet, and bake 15 minutes. They can also be frozen after baking.

RECIPE FOR SUCCESS

These bites make a great "bread" to eat with salad. Just be sure to know your carb budget for the day, as they are almost too good to stop eating! Package a portion size in a small baggie and take it along for an afternoon pick-me-up snack. The kids will love being treated to these and sliced fruit after school.

Party Cheese Log

Yield:	Serving size:	Prep time:	Cook time:
6 servings	4 slices	20 minutes plus chill time	None

Each serving has:		
3 g carbohydrate	1 g fiber	14 g protein

1 (8-oz.) pkg. cream cheese

8 oz. cheddar cheese or crumbled blue cheese, grated

¼ cup onion, grated

1 TB. Worcestershire sauce

3 TB. unsweetened cranapple juice

¼ cup dried beef, shredded

¼ cup pecans, finely chopped

1. Mix together cream cheese, cheddar cheese, onion, Worcestershire sauce, cranapple juice, and beef. Shape into a log, cover with foil, and refrigerate until firm. Just before serving, roll in pecans. Or if preferred, pecans can be mixed into log before shaping.

2. Slice into 24 pieces.

Spinach Artichoke Dip

Yield:	Serving size:	Prep time:	Cook time:
12 servings	¼ cup	10 minutes	6 minutes

Each serving has:		
3 g carbohydrate	2 g fiber	9 g protein

2 (10-oz.) pkg. frozen spinach, defrosted

½ cup green onions, chopped

1 (8-oz.) pkg. cream cheese

1 cup sour cream

¼ cup Parmesan cheese

1 (14-oz.) can artichoke hearts, drained and cut

Freshly ground black pepper to taste

2 to 3 drops hot sauce or ½ tsp. cayenne

2 cups Monterey Jack cheese, shredded

1. Cook spinach and drain well; squeeze out excess moisture with white paper towels.

2. In a microwave-safe serving dish, combine spinach, onions, cream cheese, sour cream, Parmesan cheese, artichoke hearts, pepper, and hot sauce; mix well.

3. Microwave 4 minutes, sprinkle with Monterey Jack cheese, and cook 2 minutes longer or until cheese melts.

4. Serve with vegetable scoopers.

RECIPE FOR SUCCESS

This is a favorite appetizer at many restaurants served with high-carb chips. You can serve a delectable platter of a variety of raw vegetables in various shapes and sizes knowing you are enhancing your vitamin intake plus enjoying a variety of flavors.

The Least You Need to Know

- Traditional appetizers are low carb, but at today's parties, appetizers are often high carb.
- Eat appetizers before meals, or enjoy a whole meal by consuming several.
- Take along low-carb, high-protein appetizers to parties so you aren't tempted by high-carb choices.
- Appetizers take the edge off your hunger, making it easier to eat a normal-size meal.

Snacks

Chapter 18

In This Chapter

- The appeal of snacks
- Timing your snacks
- Snacking with conscious attentiveness

Yes, it's time for a snack. We all love snacks. Whether we eat them in the late afternoon as a pick-me-up or for an energy boost during challenging outdoor activities, snacks are a very real part of most everyone's eating.

You may have been told to avoid snacking if you're watching your weight. You know how hard that is … and how unnatural. The good news is that you can have your snacks provided you budget them into your overall daily carbohydrate budget. Just follow the general guidelines found in Chapter 1. To put it another way, you can have your snacks … and eat them, too.

Your Biology Loves Snacks

It's great to think that we only need three square meals a day. Very few of us, though, eat only three meals a day. Instead, many of us eat anywhere from three to six times a day.

Snacking comes naturally. Sometimes it's because our stomach growls are calling out to be heard and satisfied. Other times, it's because our stressful lives just naturally lead us into temptation whether we are hungry or not. Or our sweet tooth takes over our brains until it has been indulged. Snacks, either junk food prepackaged versions or healthier fare, are how we satisfy these needs.

Over the past 15 years, the concept of "grazing" has become quite popular. The idea was to eat continually throughout the day, as a ruminating animal does. Grazing doesn't quite work for us humans, though. For grazing to be effective, we would need 4 stomachs, just like those cows and sheep have. Grazing doesn't fit in well with our social norms and can easily lead to overeating.

Snacking works. That's why we do it. The ideal of three-meals-and-only-three-meals-a-day is too rigorous. The shoe, so to speak, doesn't fit. Instead, let's accept the fact that snacking is here to stay and make allowances for it.

Use snacks as a way to tide you over between meals. That way, you don't get terrifically hungry and perhaps spiral out of eating—and carbohydrate—control. This chapter gives several healthy, low-carb options that will keep your sweet tooth and afternoon hunger pangs at bay.

Snacking is harmful to your weight and health if you have a bad habit of snacking throughout the day without any regard to your need for food. That's simply a bad habit and one to stop. Snacking is also harmful to your weight and health if you snack just because you are bored or if you snack mindlessly, not noticing what or how a food item gets from the refrigerator into your mouth.

But mindful, conscious snacking is just fine. That way you are aware you're eating, you are enjoying the food, and you are making sure you're staying within your daily carbohydrate allotment.

The Best Low-Carb Snacks

It's easy to find snack foods—way too easy! They're everywhere, in the grocery store, the convenience store, the vending machine, and your co-worker's desk. And how easy they are to prepare! With a few deft movements of your fingers, the wrapper comes right off and, violà, you've messed up your low-carb eating plan for the day!

The best low-carb snacks require a little forethought, planning, and preparation. They contain valuable nutrition that gives you the energy and sustenance to hold you until your next meal. They provide the most benefits when eaten slowly with conscious attentiveness, so that you enjoy the total experience.

A good snack contains low-carb foods such as nuts, meat or fish, vegetables, or fruit. They are rich-tasting enough so you can eat them sparingly, and yet you obtain enough food value to tide you over until your next meal.

TABLE TALK

Many of the snack recipes in this chapter are tote-bag tested—that is, designed to take along with you. Most don't require refrigeration, although a few do. You can put them into a snack bag or small plastic container in the morning and carry them around in your briefcase or handbag. When you need a snack during the day, you can eat them at room temperature. They don't need to be warmed or cooked.

Already Ready

The time to start thinking of preparing snacks isn't when you need one. You should have them around just in case. If you have something prepared, you won't be tempted to eat a high-carb convenience food when you get hungry.

Schedule some time now to prepare Beef Jerky and Spiced Nuts and Seeds (see recipes later in this chapter). Have the ingredients for trail mix on hand so you can put it together quickly for outings and vacations.

Rosemary Walnuts

Yield:	Serving size:	Prep time:	Cook time:
20 servings	¼ cup	5 minutes	15 minutes
Each serving has:			
1 g carbohydrate	2 g fiber	5 g protein	

6 TB. butter

1 TB. dried rosemary, crushed

1 TB. salt

½ tsp. cayenne

4 cups walnut halves

1. Preheat the oven to 325°F.

2. Melt butter in a large saucepan. Remove from heat, and add rosemary, salt, and cayenne. Add walnuts and toss gently but well. Place walnuts in a shallow roasting pan in a single layer.

3. Bake until richly brown, about 10 to 15 minutes, shaking occasionally. These nuts are nicest served warm.

RECIPE FOR SUCCESS

Nuts are a delicious snack containing hard-to-get healthy fat. You can eat them plain or toasted or even add just a couple spices to really jazz them up.

Pork on a Stick

Yield:	Serving size:	Prep time:	Cook time:
4 servings	3 skewers	30 minutes plus 4 hours chill time	5 to 8 minutes

Each serving has:		
4 g carbohydrate	2 g fiber	40 g protein

1 lb. lean, boneless, center-cut pork loin

½ cup red wine vinegar

2 TB. olive oil

1 clove garlic, minced

¼ tsp. fresh oregano, chopped fine, or ¼ tsp. dry, crushed

12 bamboo sticks

½ cup peanut butter

¼ tsp. crushed red pepper

1. Cut pork across grain into 3 × 1 × ¼-inch strips. Mix vinegar, olive oil, garlic, and oregano. Pour over pork. Refrigerate 4 hours to overnight.

2. Soak bamboo sticks 20 minutes in water. Drain pork and save marinade. Thread pork onto sticks. Grill 5 to 8 minutes on medium-high gas or charcoal grill, and brush with marinade.

3. To make sauce, warm peanut butter in a small pan with crushed red pepper. Serve hot or cold with pork on sticks.

RECIPE FOR SUCCESS

This recipe is a great way to get complete protein when you're on the run. It's ideal for snacks, lunch boxes, and even for dinner. The peanut sauce simply sparkles.

Chicken Liver Pâté with Green Pickles

Yield:	Serving size:	Prep time:	Cook time:
8 servings	1 slice	20 minutes plus chill time	15 minutes

Each serving has:		
2 g carbohydrate	1 g fiber	15 g protein

½ cup butter (1 stick)

1 lb. chicken livers

1 medium onion, chopped

½ tsp. dried thyme

½ tsp. dried rosemary

1 bay leaf

12 large white mushrooms, chopped

¼ cup brandy

½ tsp. salt

⅛ tsp. freshly ground black pepper

10 sprigs fresh parsley

16 small green dill pickles (gherkins)

1. In a large skillet, melt butter. Add chicken livers and onion. Stir over medium heat about 10 minutes. Add thyme, rosemary, bay leaf, and mushrooms. Stir frequently while cooking for 5 minutes.

2. Discard bay leaf, and pour mixture into a blender. Pour in brandy, salt, and pepper. Blend 2 minutes and then pour into a 2-cup soufflé dish. Chill.

3. Garnish with parsley. Serve with gherkins. *Note:* This dish can be covered and stored in the refrigerator for up to a week.

RECIPE FOR SUCCESS

Believe it or not, a slice of this pâté is the perfect pick-me-up for late-afternoon fatigue. It resets your energy levels and seems to soothe the adrenaline surges. But it is good any time—and that also means for breakfast.

Spiced Nuts and Seeds

Yield:	Serving size:	Prep time:	Cook time:
8 servings	¼ cup	5 minutes	5 minutes

Each serving has:		
2 g carbohydrate	2 g fiber	5 g protein

½ cup sunflower seeds

½ cup Spanish peanuts

½ cup toasted pumpkin seeds

1 tsp. chili powder

¼ tsp. cumin

⅛ tsp. garlic powder

⅛ tsp. cayenne

1. Heat sunflower seeds, peanuts, pumpkin seeds, chili powder, cumin, garlic powder, and cayenne in a skillet for about 5 minutes. Stir frequently.

Pickled Eggs

Yield:	Serving size:	Prep time:	Cook time:
6 servings	1 egg	15 minutes plus at least 24 hours chill time	10 minutes

Each serving has:		
0 g carbohydrate	0 g fiber	6 g protein

1 cup white vinegar

½ cup water

1 TB. pickling spices

2 pieces fresh ginger root, cut into ¼-in. slices

½ tsp. salt

1 clove garlic

6 hard-boiled eggs, peeled

1. Boil together vinegar, water, pickling spices, ginger root, salt, and garlic for 10 minutes.

2. Place eggs in a jar, and cover with spiced vinegar liquid. Refrigerate at least 24 hours before eating.

Beef Jerky

Yield:	Serving size:	Prep time:	Cook time:
10 servings	3 ounces	20 minutes plus overnight marinating time	7 hours

Each serving has:		
1 g carbohydrate	0 g fiber	16 g protein

2 lb. lean meat, such as brisket, flank steak, or elk steaks

$\frac{1}{2}$ cup red wine vinegar

$1\frac{1}{2}$ tsp. salt

$1\frac{1}{2}$ tsp. onion salt

$\frac{1}{2}$ tsp. freshly ground black pepper

$\frac{1}{2}$ tsp. garlic, minced

$\frac{1}{4}$ cup soy sauce

$\frac{1}{2}$ cup Worcestershire sauce

1. Place meat in freezer for one hour. Remove from freezer and slice meat as thinly as possible. Place meat in a zipper-lock plastic bag with vinegar, salt, onion salt, pepper, garlic, soy sauce, and Worcestershire sauce. Marinate overnight in the refrigerator. It is fine to marinate longer, as meat will get more tender.

2. On day of cooking, preheat the oven to 150°F.

3. Drain meat. Place on the oven racks in a single layer. Place foil on the bottom of the oven to catch any drippings.

4. Leave the oven door ajar, and bake for about 7 hours until meat is chewy and/or brittle. Store in an airtight container in the refrigerator. Jerky can be safely kept for 6 months—if you can make it last that long.

RECIPE FOR SUCCESS

Here's what to take with you when protein-rich foods won't be readily available. Take this on the airplane and on car trips. Take it hiking or anywhere you are going to want a high-protein snack when chances are good that the only snack you can get is filled with carbs.

Cheesy Nuts

Yield:	Serving size:	Prep time:	Cook time:
6 servings	1 cup	10 minutes	5 to 10 minutes
Each serving has:			
1 g carbohydrate	1 g fiber	6 g protein	

1 cup walnut halves	2 TB. Parmesan cheese
2 TB. butter	½ tsp. garlic salt

1. Preheat the oven to 350°F.

2. Boil nuts in water for 5 minutes. Drain on a paper towel. Spread nuts in a shallow baking dish. Dot with butter. Mix cheese and garlic salt with nuts. Roast for 5 minutes or more, stirring every 2 minutes to mix in butter.

Trail Mix

Yield:	Serving size:	Prep time:	Cook time:
15 servings	3 ¾ cups	10 minutes	10 to 15 minutes

Each serving has:			
6 g carbohydrate	2 g fiber	4 g protein	

4 TB. butter

½ cup sunflower seeds

½ cup pumpkin seeds

½ cup pistachio nuts, shelled

½ cup almonds

½ cup pecan halves

½ cup flaked unsweetened coconut

1 tsp. salt

¼ cup raisins

¼ cup dates, cut into quarters

¼ cup dried apricots, cut into quarters

1. Preheat the oven to 350°F.

2. Melt butter in a large, shallow, glass baking dish. Place sunflower seeds, pumpkin seeds, pistachios, almonds, pecans, and coconut in the dish. Stir to coat nuts. Sprinkle with salt.

3. Toast in the oven for 10 to 15 minutes, stirring occasionally. Remove from the oven and let cool. Then add raisins, dates, and apricots.

4. Store in the refrigerator.

Variation: You can make several substitutions to this recipe without changing the carb count very much. You can use pine nuts, cashews, and sesame seeds. You can use currants and dried figs in place of the raisins, dates, or apricots. But be careful. If you add chocolate morsels or wheat-, corn-, or rice-based foods, the carb count increases.

RECIPE FOR SUCCESS

Carry trail mix with you for hiking and outdoor adventures. The salt in the nuts can help replenish body salt lost to sweating. And the trail mix itself can give you an energy boost.

Avocado-Turkey Wrap

Yield:	Serving size:	Prep time:	Cook time:
6 servings	2 wraps	10 minutes	None

Each serving has:		
3 g carbohydrate	3 g fiber	10 g protein

12 thin (1-oz.) slices turkey breast	Pickle relish
1½ cups avocados, mashed	Jalapeños peppers, chopped
Optional toppings:	Green chilies, chopped
Capers	Nuts
Olives, chopped	Spices
Pimientos	

1. Lay out 1 slice turkey. Top with 2 tablespoons avocado, sprinkle on chosen seasonings and wrap securely. If needed, secure with toothpick.

2. Refrigerate until ready to serve.

RECIPE FOR SUCCESS

These wraps may be made with any of your favorite thinly sliced meats and rolled around fruits as well as avocados. They make great snacks as well as accompaniments to soups and salads. Make a few extras for an easy breakfast on the run.

Eggplant Crisps for Dips

Yield:	Serving size:	Prep time:	Cook time:
6 servings	3 to 4 each, depending on size of eggplant	15 minutes	8 minutes

Each serving has:		
1 g carbohydrate	1 g fiber	1 g protein

3 cups (3 small or 2 large eggplants) eggplant, peeled and cut into ¼-in. slices	2 TB. seasonings of choice—garlic powder, dill, etc.
¼ cup olive oil	Salt and freshly ground black pepper to taste

1. Preheat the oven to 425°F.

2. Coat all sides of eggplant with oil, and sprinkle with seasonings, salt, and pepper. Lightly oil a baking sheet pan, and place eggplant slices in a single layer. Bake until browned, about 8 minutes, turning once.

RECIPE FOR SUCCESS

You can make these using zucchini slices; slice the zucchini the long way and then cut to size for larger scoopers, making them easier to dip. Make extras and keep in a closed container for munching.

Variation: If you have room in your allotted carb count for the day, you can dip vegetable slices into milk and then into breadcrumbs before baking.

Homemade Peanut Butter

Yield:	Serving size:	Prep time:	Cook time:
8 servings	2 tablespoons	6 minutes	None
Each serving has:			
4 g carbohydrate	4 g fiber	12 g protein	

1 lb. roasted peanuts, unshelled, unsalted, or 2½ cups shelled

1. Shell peanuts, if necessary, and place nuts in a food processor. Process 3 minutes, stopping to scrape down sides as needed. Store in the refrigerator to keep oil from separating.

RECIPE FOR SUCCESS

How more natural can you get? This is a great treat for the kids to prepare with a bit of adult supervision. There are certainly no added preservatives, sugar, or salt in this peanut butter! Use this method with any nuts to create a variety of nut butters.

Spinach Wrappers

Yield:	Serving size:	Prep time:	Cook time:
6 servings	4 wrappers	10 minutes	None

Each serving has:		
3 g carbohydrate	1 g fiber	7 g protein

2 cups spinach leaves

2 (8-oz.) pkg. cream cheese, softened

2 TB. dried herbs of choice—dill, oregano, basil, etc.

1 TB. garlic, minced

Freshly ground black pepper to taste

½ cup pecans, finely chopped

1. Wash and dry spinach. Separate leaves and trim stems. Combine cream cheese, herbs, garlic, pepper, and pecans. Spread 1 tablespoon cream cheese mixture on 1 spinach leaf, roll, and secure with a toothpick. Stack on a platter and refrigerate until serving time.

Toasted Pumpkin Seeds

Yield:	Serving size:	Prep time:	Cook time:
6 servings	2 tablespoons	10 minutes plus ½ hour soaking time	10 minutes

Each serving has:		
2 g carbohydrate	0 g fiber	3 g protein

¾ cup seeds pulled from pumpkin

Salt water (1 TB. for 2 cups)

1. Preheat the oven to 350°F.

2. Wash seeds and remove all fibers. Prepare salt water, and soak seeds at least 30 minutes. Drain and pat seeds dry, then spread on an oiled baking sheet. Bake for 8 to 10 minutes or until golden. Watch carefully so as not to burn; they might need to be stirred so they don't stick to the pan.

3. Remove from pan, cool, and sprinkle with additional salt, if desired.

RECIPE FOR SUCCESS

This has always been one of the best things about carving the jack-o-lantern—getting to pull out the seeds and toast them for a snack after Jack was shining bright. They make great additions to salads and meat wraps as well as for eating from your hand.

Stuffed Veggies

Yield:	Serving size:	Prep time:	Cook time:
6 servings	¼ cup	15 minutes	None

Each serving has:		
5 g carbohydrate	2 g fiber	5 g protein

1 (8-oz.) pkg. cream cheese, softened

¼ cup sour cream

1 to 2 tsp. seasonings of choice—dill; horseradish; garlic powder; red pepper; radishes; or cilantro, olives, or chilies, chopped

¼ cup seafood or meat of choice—finely chopped tuna, salmon, ham, beef, turkey (optional)

6 vegetables for stuffing such as celery sticks, cucumber boats, zucchini boats, bell pepper strips, carrot sticks, tomato scoops, jicama sticks or rounds, turnip rounds, or red leaf or green leaf lettuce leaves

1. Prepare stuffing by combining cream cheese and sour cream. Add 1 teaspoon each of 2 to 3 seasonings of choice and mix well. Add seafood or meat of choice. *Note:* the base is easier to stuff or spread onto vegetables if softened at room temperature.

2. Prepare vegetable dippers by washing and peeling vegetables of choice. Cut into dipping sticks or round circles. You can make tomato scoops by hollowing out the inside of tiny red tomatoes and filling them with cream cheese mixture. You can also use lettuce leaves to fill with cream cheese mixture and roll up as finger food.

3. Vegetables can be stuffed in advance and stored in a covered container for quick, healthy snacks.

TABLE TALK

Add in carb counts for vegetables you use. The rule of thumb for quick calculations is to count an average of 5 grams carb for each 1 cup fresh vegetables. The rule of thumb for quick fiber calculations is to count an average of 2 grams fiber for each 1 cup raw fresh vegetables.

RECIPE FOR SUCCESS

This recipe has unlimited variations! Make up small containers of the cream cheese base with various seasonings. Prepare several vegetables and refrigerate them in cold water to keep crisp. The tomato scoops can be wrapped in damp paper towels to store in the refrigerator till needed. Stuff long celery stalks with filling and stick together with fillings touching, roll tightly in waxed paper; chill and cut into ½-inch pieces to serve.

The Least You Need to Know

- Eating snacks is a natural part of today's living and eating.
- Keep low-carb foods on hand for when it's time for a snack.
- Take snacks with you for outings, vacations, work, and travel.
- Use snacks as a way to manage your hunger between meals.

Vegetable Side Dishes

In This Chapter

- The joys of vegetables in low-carb eating
- Delicious varieties and tastes
- The Big Five every day

How many times have you been told to "eat your vegetables"? About a million, right? As far back as you can remember, you have heard it from your anxious parents, your doctor, dieting authorities, and every other health practitioner you've ever met. Heck, you've even been encouraged to eat your veggies by Mr. Rogers, Big Bird, and Mickey Mouse! Most likely, you've even told your own children to eat their vegetables, too.

Well, there's good reason veggies have such a powerful fan club. Of all the foods, vegetables work the hardest per ounce to keep us healthy. They offer vitamins, minerals, antioxidants, and plenty of fiber. In this chapter, we give you another good reason to eat your vegetables: they taste great!

Not Just Broccoli

Mentioning the word *vegetable* often elicits memories of the least-appealing one a person's ever eaten. Very few people wax poetic about broccoli and certainly not about brussels sprouts. But given a chance, these powerful vegetables can deliver amazing *gustatory* satisfaction.

Take a slow and observant walk down the produce aisle of your grocery store. You may be amazed. You'll likely see vegetables whose names are complete mysteries to you, and you may not know what to do with them! So get ready! These recipes will expand your vegetable-cooking repertoire to include a wider variety of delicious vegetables, even ones with such names as *celeriac* and *jicama*.

Gustatory means relating to or associated with the sense of taste. Gustatory satisfaction pleases your taste buds and delights your whole sensation of taste.

TABLE TALK

Green vegetables are the workhorses of the vegetable world because they consistently deliver excellent nutrition for very few carbohydrates. For instance, the carb count for ½ cup cooked broccoli is about 4 grams.

The Big Five

No, the "Big Five" isn't a new athletic conference; it's that magic number of fruits and vegetables we are all supposed to eat each and every day. Eating up to 10 servings is even better.

Let's face it, if you're on a low-carb eating plan for your weight, diabetes, or other aspects of your health or appearance, you care about feeling good and looking good. Eating those 5 to 10 servings accelerates your success. You'll actually feel better and likely have more energy—two things that go a long way to helping you stick with a low-carb eating plan.

Vegetables offer healthy carbs and are often high in fiber. Don't pass up eating vegetables because you're saving your carbs for white and fluffy high-carb treats. The low and modest amount of carbs in vegetables feed your health and well-being. Think of them as "feel-good" foods.

Don't think of a serving of a vegetable as a giant mound of something green. Our habit of thinking of servings as some gargantuan portion is what gets a lot of us in weight trouble in the first place. A serving size of vegetables is usually about ½ cup cooked vegetables and 1 cup raw. A good-size salad is often 2 servings. It's really quite easy to eat three modest servings at dinner or lunch.

The list of green vegetables is long—green beans, lettuces, broccoli, spinach, kale, collard greens, celery, fennel, brussels sprouts, cabbage, asparagus, parsley, and many others.

Think of all those vegetables in the produce section just waiting for you to take them home and try them out. Some already are your good friends, but some you have passed by week after week for years. Why not take one home and try it as a side dish? Experiment, and you may find another delicious new friend for life.

Brussels Sprouts with Pecans

Yield:	Serving size:	Prep time:	Cook time:
6 servings	1/6 recipe	20 minutes	10 minutes

Each serving has:		
4 g carbohydrate	6 g fiber	3 g protein

1/4 tsp. salt

1 lb. brussels sprouts, trimmed

3 TB. butter

1/4 cup pecans, chopped

Freshly ground black pepper

1. To a large saucepan of boiling water, add salt and brussels sprouts. Cover and cook until tender, about 10 minutes. Drain, place in a shallow serving dish, and cover to keep warm.

2. In a small saucepan, melt butter over medium heat. Cook until brown. Add pecans and toss until lightly browned. Pour over brussels sprouts and sprinkle with pepper to taste.

RECIPE FOR SUCCESS

This cruciferous vegetable takes well to just plain butter. Add in the sautéed pecans, and you'll find that this is a side dish you love.

Warm Caraway Cabbage with Carrots

Yield:	Serving size:	Prep time:	Cook time:
8 servings	3/4 cup	15 minutes	12 minutes

Each serving has:		
9 g carbohydrate	2 g fiber	1 g protein

1 TB. butter

8 cups mixed green and red shredded cabbage and carrots

1 1/4 tsp. caraway seeds

1/3 cup golden raisins

3 TB. cider vinegar

1/4 cup water

Salt and freshly ground black pepper

1. In a large, shallow skillet, heat butter over high heat. Add cabbage mixture, and stir-fry until just wilted, 2 to 3 minutes. Add caraway seeds, raisins, and vinegar. Stir-fry 1 minute. Add water, and continue cooking over high heat, stirring occasionally, until most of the water is absorbed and cabbage is cooked, about 8 minutes. Season with salt and pepper to taste. Serve immediately.

Fennel and Tomatoes

Yield:	Serving size:	Prep time:	Cook time:
8 servings	⅛ recipe	20 minutes	30 minutes
Each serving has:			
6 g carbohydrate	3 g fiber	2 g protein	

3 medium fennel bulbs (about 2 lb.)

2 TB. butter

1 medium onion, finely chopped

2 medium tomatoes, seeded and chopped

¼ tsp. dried thyme

¼ cup water

Salt and freshly ground black pepper

1. Trim stems and bottoms from fennel bulbs. Chop fronds from stems, reserve 2 tablespoons, and discard stems. Chop fronds and set aside. Chop bulbs and cook in boiling salted water 2 to 3 minutes. Drain and set aside.

2. In a medium saucepan, melt butter over medium-low heat. Add onion and cook until just browned, 5 to 10 minutes. Add tomatoes, thyme, water, and cooked fennel. Cover and cook over low heat until tender, about 25 minutes.

3. Remove cover and cook until liquid evaporates, 3 to 5 minutes. Increase heat to medium, and cook 2 minutes. Season with salt and pepper to taste.

4. Place in a serving dish, and garnish with reserved chopped fennel fronds. Serve immediately.

RECIPE FOR SUCCESS

Fennel goes well with any main dish, from beef to seafood. If you haven't yet eaten this vegetable, try it—you may just fall in love.

Spaghetti Squash with Italian Sauce

Yield:	Serving size:	Prep time:	Cook time:
8 servings	$\frac{1}{8}$ squash and $\frac{1}{8}$ sauce	20 minutes	1 hour plus 5 minutes

Each serving has:		
14 g carbohydrate	2 g fiber	7 g protein

1 (3 lb.) spaghetti squash

2 TB. olive oil

1 TB. butter

1 (8-oz.) pkg. fresh mushrooms, sliced

2 medium tomatoes, chopped

1 medium zucchini, diced

5 green onions, including tops, chopped

1 tsp. garlic, minced

1 medium red bell pepper, cored, seeded, and cut into $\frac{1}{8}$-in. strips

$\frac{1}{2}$ tsp. dried oregano

Salt and freshly ground black pepper to taste

$\frac{3}{4}$ cup freshly grated Parmesan cheese

1. Preheat the oven to 350°F.

2. Bake whole squash 1 hour or until tender when pierced with fork. Remove from the oven and allow to cool 5 to 10 minutes. Halve lengthwise and remove seeds. With a fork, pull out spaghetti-like strands, and place in a large serving bowl. Set aside.

3. In a large skillet, heat oil and butter over medium heat. Add mushrooms, tomatoes, zucchini, green onions, garlic, bell pepper, and oregano. Cook until soft, 4 to 5 minutes. Pour mixture over squash, and toss to combine. Add salt and pepper to taste. Sprinkle with Parmesan cheese, and serve immediately.

Variation: Use spaghetti squash as a substitute for spaghetti or pasta in any recipe. The carbohydrate count of 1 cup cooked wheat spaghetti is about 40 grams. The same amount of cooked spaghetti squash is only 10 grams. The squash also contains more nutrients, plus each serving counts toward your five or more fruits and vegetables per day.

RECIPE FOR SUCCESS

Spaghetti squash's mild flavor blends well with the stronger tastes of Italian cuisine. Enjoy the spaghetti squash in this recipe as a hearty side dish with a meat entrée, or serve it plain with other Italian sauces, such as Alfredo or meat sauce.

Green Peas Cooked in Lettuce

Yield:	Serving size:	Prep time:	Cook time:
6 servings	About ²/₃ cup	15 minutes	10 minutes

Each serving has:			
9 g carbohydrate	5 g fiber	5 g protein	

3½ cups frozen peas

4 TB. butter

3 green onions, chopped

4 Bibb lettuce leaves, cut in half

Salt and freshly ground black pepper to taste

1. Steam peas over boiling water for 5 minutes until partially cooked.

2. In a heavy skillet, sauté 2 tablespoons butter with green onions and lettuce. Sprinkle with salt and pepper, cover, and cook on low for 3 to 4 minutes. Add partially cooked peas to the skillet, and cook over low heat an additional 3 minutes.

3. Transfer to a serving dish, and top with remaining 2 tablespoons butter.

Variation: Substitute snow peas or sugar snap peas for the green peas in this recipe. You can also top with mint or minced fresh ginger root, or even sprinkle with toasted sesame seeds.

RECIPE FOR SUCCESS

This recipe is a simple, yet interesting side dish for meats and fish. If you've never cooked lettuce before, you will find that it softly enhances the flavor of the peas.

Colorful Broccoli

Yield:	Serving size:	Prep time:	Cook time:
6 servings	About ²/₃ cup	20 minutes	18 minutes

Each serving has:		
9 g carbohydrate	6 g fiber	5 g protein

1½ lb. broccoli, cut into florets

2 carrots, sliced

1 TB. butter

½ tsp. garlic, minced

½ cup water

1 tsp. dried basil

⅛ tsp. cayenne

8 oz. *jicama*, peeled and cut into thin strips

3 plum tomatoes, cut into wedges

2 TB. grated Parmesan cheese

1. Steam broccoli and carrots until tender. Drain. In a heavy skillet, heat butter. Sauté garlic. Add basil and cayenne and cook about 2 minutes. Add broccoli and carrots. Heat thoroughly. Add jicama and tomatoes and mix. Remove to a serving dish. Sprinkle with Parmesan, and serve right away.

DEFINITION

Jicama is a root vegetable used in Mexican cuisine. It has a fresh and slightly sweet (though bland) taste. Along with the other vegetables, it adds a full rainbow of nutrients, vitamins, and antioxidants. Colorful Broccoli is an excellent accompaniment to any main course dish.

Southwestern Vegetables

Yield:	Serving size:	Prep time:	Cook time:
15 servings	$\frac{1}{12}$ recipe	20 minutes	20 minutes

Each serving has:		
19 g carbohydrate	6 g fiber	8 g protein

1 clove garlic, minced

2 TB. butter

1 (16-oz.) can corn, drained

3 medium tomatoes, chopped

2 medium zucchini, sliced $\frac{1}{4}$-in. thick

$\frac{1}{4}$ tsp. cumin

1 (15-oz.) can black beans, drained

$\frac{1}{2}$ tsp. salt

$\frac{1}{4}$ tsp. freshly ground black pepper

$\frac{1}{4}$ cup fresh cilantro, chopped

3 TB. pine nuts

1. Sauté garlic in butter over medium-high heat until fragrant. Add corn, tomatoes, zucchini, cumin, beans, salt, and pepper; mix well. Sauté for 10 to 15 minutes. Remove to serving dish. Sprinkle with cilantro and pine nuts and serve warm.

Asparagus with Hollandaise Sauce

Yield:	Serving size:	Prep time:	Cook time:
6 servings	$\frac{1}{6}$ recipe	10 minutes	6 minutes

Each serving has:		
1 g carbohydrate	2 g fiber	4 g protein

$\frac{1}{2}$ cup butter (1 stick)

4 large egg yolks

1 TB. lemon juice

Freshly ground black pepper to taste

1 lb. fresh asparagus

1. Heat butter in the microwave until just melted. Put egg yolks, lemon juice, and pepper into a blender. Slowly pour in melted butter, and blend for several seconds.

2. Steam asparagus spears over boiling water until tender. Remove to serving platter and top with hollandaise sauce.

Ginger Carrots

Yield:	Serving size:	Prep time:	Cook time:
6 servings	⅙ recipe	10 minutes	5 minutes

Each serving has:		
5 g carbohydrate	2 g fiber	1 g protein

1 lb. baby carrots

3 TB. butter

1 tsp. ground ginger

1 tsp. honey

¼ tsp. salt

¼ tsp. coarsely ground fresh black pepper

1. Steam carrots briefly until they are *al dente*.

2. In a large, heavy skillet, melt butter over medium heat. Add ginger, honey, and steamed carrots, and stir gently to coat thoroughly. Add salt and pepper.

DEFINITION

Al dente is an Italian term that indicates a stage of doneness in both pasta and vegetables. The food is cooked to the point before it becomes mushy or too soft. Al dente food has some crunch left.

Green Beans, Pecans, and Feta

Yield:	Serving size:	Prep time:	Cook time:
6 servings	⅙ recipe	15 minutes	5 minutes

Each serving has:		
5 g carbohydrate	5 g fiber	5 g protein

1½ lb. fresh string beans, trimmed and cut into 1-in. pieces

¾ cup olive oil

1 tsp. dried basil

⅓ cup white wine vinegar

½ tsp. garlic, minced

¼ tsp. salt

¼ tsp. freshly ground black pepper

½ cup pecans, coarsely chopped

½ cup crumbled feta cheese

½ cup red bell pepper, diced

1. Steam string beans until barely tender. In a small bowl, combine olive oil, basil, vinegar, garlic, salt, and pepper. Place beans in a shallow serving bowl. Sprinkle with pecans, feta, and red bell pepper, and toss with olive oil dressing.

Variation: Substitute other cheeses such as Parmesan, cheddar, or Swiss for the feta in this recipe.

RECIPE FOR SUCCESS

Even string beans become majestic when dressed up with pecans and feta cheese. Enjoy this recipe anytime you find the string beans looking terrific and fresh at the grocery store.

Tomatoes Stuffed with Blue Cheese and Mushrooms

Yield:	Serving size:	Prep time:	Cook time:
4 servings	1 tomato plus stuffing	20 minutes	25 minutes
Each serving has:			
5 g carbohydrate	3 g fiber	4 g protein	

4 large tomatoes
2 TB. butter
$\frac{1}{4}$ lb. white mushrooms

$\frac{1}{2}$ tsp. dried parsley
4 TB. blue cheese, crumbled

1. Preheat the oven to 350°F.

2. Cut off top of tomatoes. Take out about $\frac{1}{2}$ interior without piercing skins. Heat butter in a heavy skillet, and sauté mushrooms with parsley until tender.

3. Divide mushroom mixture, and put into tomatoes. Top with 1 tablespoon blue cheese each. Put tomatoes into a baking dish, and bake for 25 minutes or until done.

RECIPE FOR SUCCESS

Tomatoes aren't just for salads and sauces. These baked tomatoes add lots of pizzazz to simpler meat and fish dishes.

Baked Onions

Yield:	Serving size:	Prep time:	Cook time:
6 servings	1 onion	15 minutes	1 hour
Each serving has:			
8 g carbohydrate	2 g fiber	1 g protein	

6 large sweet onions, such as Vidalia	Salt and freshly ground black pepper to taste
	6 tsp. butter

1. Preheat the oven to 375°F.

2. Peel onions and place each on a foil square. Salt and pepper as desired. Score onion about halfway through. Place 1 teaspoon butter into each onion, and wrap onion well in the foil. Place in a baking pan, and bake 1 hour.

 RECIPE FOR SUCCESS

These onions can easily take the place of a baked potato without the extra carbs. Garnish with bacon bits, green onions, and sour cream, if desired.

Broccoli-Stuffed Tomatoes

Yield:	Serving size:	Prep time:	Cook time:
6 servings	1 tomato	20 minutes	35 minutes
Each serving has:			
6 g carbohydrate	3 g fiber	3 g protein	

6 large, firm tomatoes	2 TB. fresh parsley, chopped
1 TB. salt	Freshly ground black pepper to taste
2 TB. butter	
½ onion, chopped	6 TB. olive oil
1½ cups broccoli florets, chopped or 1 (10-oz.) pkg. frozen chopped broccoli	½ cup water
	6 TB. almonds, chopped

1. Wash tomatoes and cut a thin slice from stem end. Save to use later. Scoop out pulp, drain and chop pulp, and set aside. Sprinkle inside of each tomato with $\frac{1}{2}$ teaspoon salt; invert and drain.

2. In a large skillet, heat butter and sauté onions and broccoli until soft. Add parsley, pepper, and $\frac{1}{2}$ tomato pulp. Fill tomatoes with broccoli mixture, and set tomatoes in a baking pan. Replace tomato "lids," and drizzle 1 tablespoon oil over each tomato. Pour water into bottom of pan, and bake 30 minutes or until hot.

3. Carefully remove and discard tomato lid, and sprinkle tomato with chopped almonds. May serve hot or cold.

RECIPE FOR SUCCESS

Tomato cups can be filled with many different cheeses, meats, seafood, and vegetables. They make delicious holders for fresh tuna or chicken salad. You can even bake the tomatoes with vegetable salad in them for a hot luncheon on a chilly day.

This recipe is the perfect accompaniment to any meat dish. Leftovers are delicious as a cold lunch the next day or even for breakfast!

Creamed Cabbage

Yield:	Serving size:	Prep time:	Cook time:
6 servings	$\frac{1}{2}$ cup	5 minutes	20 minutes

Each serving has:			
4 g carbohydrate	1 g fiber	1 g protein	

2 TB. butter

$\frac{3}{4}$ cup onion, chopped

4 cups cabbage, sliced

$\frac{1}{2}$ cup water

$\frac{1}{2}$ cup sour cream

Salt and freshly ground black pepper to taste

Additional seasonings as desired

1. Melt butter in a skillet, and sauté onion until tender. Add cabbage and water and cover pan. Simmer for 5 minutes or until cabbage is tender. Remove cover and boil until water is gone.

2. Stir in sour cream, salt, pepper, and serve.

Green Bean Almandine

Yield:	Serving size:	Prep time:	Cook time:
6 servings	½ cup	10 minutes	20 minutes

Each serving has:		
5 g carbohydrate	5 g fiber	4 g protein

1½ lb. fresh green beans, trimmed (3 cups)

3 TB. butter

½ cup almonds, slivered

1 tsp. garlic, minced

¼ tsp. fresh rosemary, chopped or ¼ tsp. dried

Salt and freshly ground black pepper to taste

2 TB. pimiento, chopped

1. Bring water to boil in a large pot, and add green beans. Boil until just tender, about 6 to 8 minutes. Drain beans and run under cold water in a colander or plunge them into ice water to prevent further cooking. Pat beans dry, and refrigerate or set aside until ready to use.

2. Melt butter in a skillet, and sauté almonds, garlic, rosemary, salt, and pepper. Add green beans and pimiento, and stir until heated through.

RECIPE FOR SUCCESS

You can blanch the beans and refrigerate them the day before or earlier in the day. A few minutes before serving, sauté the seasonings and beans. If fresh beans are unavailable, you may substitute the long frozen beans and omit the first step of blanching. This is a quick and easy, yet elegant, side dish.

Southern Greens

Yield:	Serving size:	Prep time:	Cook time:
6 servings	½ cup	20 minutes	45 minutes

Each serving has:		
3 g carbohydrate	5 g fiber	5 g protein

2 lb. mustard greens

8¼ cups water

1 beef bouillon cube

2 slices raw bacon or 1 oz. ham, cut into small pieces

2 TB. olive oil

½ cup onion, chopped

½ tsp. garlic, minced

½ tsp. salt

1 tsp. freshly ground black pepper

1. Wash greens and tear into bite-size pieces, discarding any tough stems. In a large pot, boil 8 cups water and add greens; boil 20 minutes until tender and then drain and set aside.

2. In a cast-iron Dutch oven, bring remaining ¼ cup water to a boil, and dissolve bouillon cube. Add bacon pieces and cook. Add oil, onion, garlic, salt, and pepper. Stir in greens, and reduce heat to a low simmer.

3. Cook at least 20 minutes until greens are very tender. Stir periodically, adding water as needed to keep greens from burning.

RECIPE FOR SUCCESS

Washing fresh greens to get all the sand and grit off the leaves can be a major ordeal. Now the packaged greens make it too easy not to try this simple high-vitamin dish any time of the year. Try various greens such as turnip, mustard, collard, kale, or a mixture of several. Try cooking turnips in the same pot of greens; this gives them a wonderful flavor.

Swiss Onions

Yield:	Serving size:	Prep time:	Cook time:
8 servings	$\frac{1}{2}$ cup	15 minutes	25 minutes

Each serving has:		
11 g carbohydrate	1 g fiber	4 g protein

3 large sweet onions, such as Vidalia, quartered

2 TB. butter

1 cup (8-oz.) Swiss cheese, shredded

1 cup mayonnaise

2 TB. white wine

1 clove garlic, minced

$\frac{1}{2}$ tsp. cayenne

3 TB. fresh parsley, chopped, for garnish

1. Preheat the oven to 375°F.

2. Sauté onions in butter until tender. In a bowl, combine cheese, mayonnaise, wine, garlic, and cayenne. Toss with onions, and pour into a greased baking dish. Bake 25 minutes. Top with fresh parsley and serve.

RECIPE FOR SUCCESS

This dish is reminiscent of French onion soup. You can substitute other vegetables for the onion or cut onion amount in half; add vegetables such as green beans or broccoli.

Tasty Turnips

Yield:	Serving size:	Prep time:	Cook time:
6 servings	$\frac{1}{2}$ cup	10 minutes	20 minutes

Each serving has:		
5 g carbohydrate	1 g fiber	1 g protein

4 medium turnips

1 tsp. sugar

$\frac{1}{2}$ tsp. salt

2 cups water

2 beef bouillon cubes

1 tsp. freshly ground black pepper

4 TB. butter

1. Peel and quarter turnips, sprinkle with sugar and salt, and set aside.

2. Boil 2 cups water in a saucepan, and dissolve bouillon cubes. Add turnips, pepper, and additional water to just cover turnips. Cover pot, and simmer until turnips are tender, about 15 minutes. Watch carefully, adding additional water if needed.

3. Drain turnips and toss with butter. Mash or leave in pieces as desired.

RECIPE FOR SUCCESS

Turnips are a wonderful substitute for potatoes. When they are mashed with lots of butter, you can hardly tell they are not potatoes. The sugar keeps the turnips from tasting bitter. Turnips are also delicious cooked in the same pot with Southern Greens (see recipe earlier in chapter).

Vibrant Peppers and Tomatoes

Yield:	Serving size:	Prep time:	Cook time:
12 servings	½ bell pepper	20 minutes	35 minutes

Each serving has:		
4 g carbohydrate	2 g fiber	1 g protein

3 red bell peppers

3 yellow bell peppers

¼ cup olive oil

3 cloves garlic, minced

24 red cherry tomatoes

24 yellow cherry tomatoes, or if unavailable, substitute more red cherry or grape tomatoes

3 TB. drained capers

2 TB. fresh thyme leaves

Salt and freshly ground black pepper to taste

½ cup balsamic vinegar

½ cup water

1. Preheat the oven to 425°F.

2. Cut red and yellow bell peppers in half lengthwise, and remove core and seeds. Keep peppers intact as they will be holders for other vegetables. Oil a large baking pan, and stand peppers up in the pan. Brush peppers with oil.

3. Divide garlic among peppers, sprinkling into bottom of each pepper. Place 2 red cherry tomatoes and 2 yellow cherry tomatoes into each pepper, and sprinkle with capers, thyme, salt, and pepper. Drizzle each filled pepper with oil.

4. Pour about ¼ cup water into the bottom of the pan. Bake 35 minutes, and cool to room temperature. Serve ½ pepper on each plate, drizzled lightly with balsamic vinegar.

RECIPE FOR SUCCESS

This is the perfect dish for a BBQ or any buffet meal. Layer anchovies into the bottom of each pepper for additional flavor, or spice them up with a few slices of pickled jalapeño peppers.

Yellow Squash Casserole

Yield:	Serving size:	Prep time:	Cook time:
6 servings	½ cup	10 minutes	30 minutes
Each serving has:			
12 g carbohydrate	3 g fiber	5 g protein	

2 lb. fresh yellow crookneck squash	2 TB. butter or olive oil
Water	1 onion, chopped
¼ tsp. salt	½ bell pepper, chopped
1 cup Basic Cream Soup (see recipe in Chapter 14)	2 carrots, chopped
1 large egg, beaten	1 TB. fresh parsley, chopped
1 (3-oz.) pkg. cream cheese, softened	1 TB. paprika
1 tsp. freshly ground black pepper	2 tomatoes, chopped, for garnish

1. Slice squash and boil in salted water until barely tender; drain and set aside. Combine soup, egg, cream cheese, and pepper; set aside.

2. In a skillet, melt butter and sauté onion, bell pepper, and carrots until tender. Mix in soup mixture and heat. When all ingredients are combined, stir in squash and remove from heat.

3. Pour into a greased baking dish, sprinkle with parsley and paprika, and bake 20 minutes. Serve with fresh chopped tomato for garnish.

Variation: You can substitute fresh or frozen okra or even brussels sprouts for the squash. This basic recipe is quite useful for most any vegetable.

RECIPE FOR SUCCESS

This recipe makes a great addition to covered dish suppers. Add cooked ground beef for a meal in itself.

The Least You Need to Know

- Vegetables add great variety and enjoyment to meals as side dishes.
- Eating your vegetables is certainly good for you and meets the requirements of low-carb eating.
- When purchasing vegetables, buy only the freshest and healthiest.
- Experiment with unfamiliar vegetables to increase your enjoyment of these health workhorses.

Side Salads

In This Chapter

- Beyond the ho-hum salad
- Naturally low-carb salads
- Attention-getting side salads
- Dressings for all tastes

It's good for you and you order it, but you seldom get excited about it. The "it" we're talking about is the side salad that's just about always included with your entrée in sit-down restaurants. Even without asking, you know what to expect: some iceberg lettuce, maybe a few pieces of a darker green leaf lettuce, a cherry tomato (if you're lucky), a couple dried croutons (if you're not), and perhaps some grated carrot or red cabbage shreds for color. Your choice of dressing usually includes ranch, blue cheese, and some kind of vinaigrette.

You can easily prepare this salad in your home—which is why you may not. Even though it's good for you, there's a good chance it holds little appeal after years and years of eating it.

So welcome to appetizing salads. In this chapter, we have included salads even our teenage boys not only eat but actually request. Salads deserve their rightful place among delicious cuisine, not among the good-for-you-but-boring foods.

The Custom of Salads

Over the centuries, people have eaten salads with meals, either before, as we do in the United States, or after, as some Europeans prefer. Salads are a customary part of feasts, fancy dinners, and virtually every meal except breakfast. Of course, you certainly can eat salad for breakfast, too. A favorite restaurant of ours offers "Breakfast Salad" as an entrée.

Folk wisdom proves right again. Today, we know the reasons why salads have stood the test of time. The ingredients in salads supply important nutrients in the form of vitamins, minerals, antioxidants, and fiber. Generally speaking, the darker, more vibrant-colored lettuces have more nutrients.

Salads are excellent as side dishes for low-carb eating. You can add a salad to any main course because salads have some carbohydrates, but not many, and they add fiber to your diet. Plus, they have a refreshing quality that lightens the meal and yet satisfies.

Salad Pizzazz

A little pizzazz can turn an otherwise ho-hum salad into a delicious treat. The first time we tasted the Fiesta Confetti Salad (see recipe later in this chapter) we were in food heaven. Enhanced with Southwestern spices of cumin and cilantro, this salad—really a modified salsa—is sure far from boring!

The wonderful Romaine Salad with Capers and Salami (also featured later in this chapter) also contains marinated artichoke hearts, anchovy paste, raisins, grated Parmesan cheese, and pine nuts. Remember, this is just a tossed lettuce salad but one tossed with remarkable ingredients that have our party guests practically licking the salad bowl.

The pizzazz in salads comes from adding unusual spices, vegetables, and even fruits to the standard tossed or vegetable salad. Meats, fish, and cheeses add depth and richness to a salad's taste. You'll find many good examples of salad pizzazz in these recipes.

Dressing Up Your Salads

Salad dressings are sneaky concoctions. We really only need a "splash" of salad dressing to enhance the flavor of lettuce and vegetables, but so often we tend to spoon on so much we hide the appealing tastes of the lettuces and vegetables. Too much dressing will also overload your fat intake for the day, so go easy with it.

Here's a basic, simple, time-tested salad dressing: put lettuce and vegetables—the greens—into a large salad bowl. Sprinkle olive oil over the greens. Toss until each leaf is coated with a thin layer of the oil. Add more oil if needed. Then add a splash or two of your favorite vinegar and toss. Taste to make sure you have enough vinegar but not too much. Add a sprinkling of salt and some freshly ground black pepper. Then add your special pizzazz to the salad such as nuts, seeds, pieces of fresh or dried fruit, shredded cheese, and marinated condiments.

The dressings in these salads are low carb and contain healthy ingredients. But when purchasing salad dressing in the store, take caution to make sure you're getting the best. Read the label to assure that the amount of carbs per tablespoon is very low.

TABLE TALK

Store lettuce unwashed in a sealed plastic bag with a small hole or two for ventilation. Place the bag in a cold area of your refrigerator, as it lasts longest and stays crispest when stored at a temperature just above 32°F.

To restore partially wilted raw vegetables and lettuce, put them into a container of cold water for several minutes. This adds moisture and increases crispness.

- The best oils for salad dressings are cold expeller-pressed oils. This method of obtaining the oil doesn't use heat. Using heat to extract the oil changes the nature of the oil and creates undesirable trans-fatty acids. Some good oils to use are walnut, olive, almond, canola, hazelnut, and flax seed. If your grocer doesn't carry cold expeller-pressed oils, find them at the health food store.

- Some dressings are made with bacon fat and are quite excellent. Animal fats, including butter, can be heated without deterioration or change in quality provided you don't burn them.

- Avoid purchasing low-fat salad dressings, as they are higher in carbohydrates and contain both added sugars and starches.

- Keep freshly bottled natural lemon or lime juice in the refrigerator for salad dressings. These are available at the health food groceries. You can also squeeze fresh lemons and limes for dressings.

- The tanginess of salad dressings comes from the vinegar or lemon/lime juice. If you like your dressing tangy, use more. If not, cut back on the vinegar or juice.

- With the exception of balsamic vinegar, vinegars contain no carbohydrates. Balsamic vinegar has 1 gram carbohydrate for 1 tablespoon.

- Add spices, herbs, and condiments for more flavor. Experiment with mustards, olives, hot or mild peppers, parsley, oregano, cayenne, balsam, cilantro, rosemary, and virtually anything else in your spice cabinet.

Romaine Salad with Capers and Salami

Yield:	Serving size:	Prep time:	Cook time:
6 servings	$\frac{1}{6}$ recipe	10 minutes	None

Each serving has:		
4 g carbohydrate	1 g fiber	3 g protein

1 head romaine lettuce, washed and torn into bite-size pieces

3 TB. olive oil

3 TB. red wine vinegar

1 TB. flax seeds

2 TB. seeds or nuts—pine nuts, pumpkin seeds, sunflower seeds, pecans, slivered almonds, chopped walnuts

1 to 2 tsp. capers or to taste

2 marinated artichoke heart pieces, cut into slices

$\frac{1}{2}$ tsp. anchovy paste

2 TB. raisins, dried cranberries, or dried cherries

2 slices of salami, thinly sliced and fried

2 TB. Parmesan cheese, shredded

2 TB. croutons

1. Spin lettuce until dry, put into a large salad bowl, and sprinkle with olive oil. Toss, making sure to lightly coat each leaf. Sprinkle with red wine vinegar and toss.

2. Add flax seeds, other seeds, capers, artichoke heart pieces, anchovy paste, raisins, salami, cheese, and croutons and toss well.

Variation: To make this into a main course salad, add $\frac{1}{2}$ pound roast beef, cut into strips.

RECIPE FOR SUCCESS

Romaine Salad with Capers and Salami is the most appealing tossed salad we know. It's even good eaten the next day. Our children who hate veggies actually want to eat this salad—we think it's because it has the very mild protein taste of the anchovy paste.

Winter Salad

Yield:	Serving size:	Prep time:	Cook time:
6 servings	⅙ salad	20 minutes	None
Each serving has:			
3 g carbohydrate	2 g fiber	2 g protein	

For salad dressing:

3 TB. fresh parsley, finely chopped

2 TB. olive oil

2 TB. walnut oil

1 TB. vinegar

1 TB. lemon juice

1 tsp. Dijon mustard

¼ tsp. salt

⅛ tsp. freshly ground black pepper

For salad:

1 (8-oz.) pkg. white mushrooms, thinly sliced

12 radishes, thinly sliced

¼ jicama, peeled and thinly sliced

4 green onions, thinly sliced by hand

1 clove garlic, minced

6 romaine lettuce leaves

1. Combine parsley, olive oil, walnut oil, vinegar, lemon juice, mustard, salt, and pepper in a screw-top jar and shake well.

2. If not using immediately, refrigerate mushrooms, radishes, and jicama in separate containers covered with plastic wrap. When ready to serve, combine with green onions, garlic, and dressing, and serve in lettuce cups.

RECIPE FOR SUCCESS

Enjoy this unusual blending of vegetables as a side dish with a heavier main course such as beef, pork, or ham.

Celery Root Salad

Yield:	Serving size:	Prep time:	Cook time:
6 servings	$\frac{1}{6}$ salad	20 minutes	1 hour

Each serving has:		
10 g carbohydrate	3 g fiber	2 g protein

1 celery root (also known as celeriac)	1 tsp. peppercorns
6 small onions, peeled	2 small bay leaves
$\frac{1}{4}$ cup dry white wine	4 TB. butter
$\frac{3}{4}$ cup chicken bouillon	$\frac{1}{4}$ tsp. salt
	$\frac{1}{4}$ tsp. paprika

1. Peel celery root, and cut into small sections like French fries. Steam for 15 minutes. Combine celery root, onions, wine, bouillon, peppercorns, bay leaves, butter, and salt in a saucepan. Simmer over low heat for 45 minutes. Remove bay leaf.

2. Cool in the refrigerator. Serve cold with a sprinkling of paprika.

Guacamole

Yield:	Serving size:	Prep time:	Cook time:
8 servings	$\frac{1}{3}$ cup	10 minutes plus 30 minutes chill time	None

Each serving has:		
2 g carbohydrate	5 g fiber	2 g protein

3 avocados, pitted	1 TB. fresh cilantro, chopped
$\frac{1}{3}$ cup lime juice	Salt and freshly ground black pepper to taste
1 large tomato, chopped	
1 clove garlic, minced	

1. Mash avocado pulp, leaving a few small lumps. Stir in lime juice, tomato, garlic, cilantro, salt, and pepper. Cover tightly and chill at least 30 minutes.

2. Serve chilled over lettuce leaf or as garnish to other foods.

Fiesta Confetti Salad

Yield:	Serving size:	Prep time:	Cook time:
24 servings	½ cup	25 minutes plus chill time	None

Each serving has:		
14 g carbohydrate	5 g fiber	5 g protein

1 green bell pepper, chopped

1 red bell pepper, chopped

2 tomatoes, chopped

1 papaya or mango, peeled, seeded, and chopped

3 green onions, chopped

1 clove garlic, minced

¼ cup fresh cilantro, chopped

1 (11-oz.) can corn, drained

1 (15-oz.) can black beans, drained and rinsed

1 (4-oz.) can green chilies

½ tsp. cumin

½ tsp. salt

½ tsp. freshly ground black pepper

1 small jalapeño pepper, minced (optional)

3 limes, sliced

1. Combine green and red bell peppers, tomatoes, papaya, green onions, garlic, cilantro, corn, beans, chilies, cumin, salt, black pepper, jalapeño (if using), and limes in a large bowl. Mix well. Chill before serving.

RECIPE FOR SUCCESS

This recipe is a delightful surprise as a salad and as a salsa. Serve with meat, Mexican entrées, chicken, and fish. Eat for lunch and also breakfast. It's totally good for you. Store salad in an air-tight container in the refrigerator for up to one week.

Five-Day Coleslaw

Yield:	Serving size:	Prep time:	Cook time:
6 servings	¾ cup or ⅙ recipe	15 minutes plus overnight chill time	5 minutes

Each serving has:			
3 g carbohydrate	2 g fiber	1 g protein	

2 cups red cabbage, thinly sliced

2 cups green cabbage, thinly sliced

½ cup celery, sliced

½ cup bell pepper, coarsely chopped

2 TB. mayonnaise

1 TB. white wine vinegar

1 TB. garlic, minced

1 TB. fresh ginger, minced or 1 tsp. ground

1 tsp. dry mustard

Salt and freshly ground black pepper to taste

1. Combine red and green cabbage, celery, bell pepper, and mayonnaise. In a small saucepan, combine vinegar, garlic, ginger, mustard, salt, and pepper and bring to a boil. Pour over vegetables and mix well.

2. Cover and refrigerate overnight before serving. Salad will keep well for 5 days covered in the refrigerator.

RECIPE FOR SUCCESS

Even though the name is "Five-Day Coleslaw" we doubt you will have any left for that long. This crunchy, low-carb salad is wonderful wrapped up in meat wraps or used as a base for grilled meat salads. It is just the thing for a pick-me-up snack in the afternoon when the desire for something crunchy hits.

Asian Spinach Salad

Yield:	Serving size:	Prep time:	Cook time:
6 servings	⅙ recipe	10 minutes	None
Each serving has:			
10 g carbohydrate	1 g fiber	7 g protein	

For salad dressing:

¼ cup soy sauce

3 TB. olive oil

1 tsp. sesame oil (hot chili oil is best)

½ tsp. molasses

For salad:

1 (10-oz.) pkg. baby spinach leaves

½ cup water chestnuts

1 (8-oz.) can bean sprouts, drained

3 hard-boiled eggs, sliced

1 TB. almonds, slivered for garnish

1 TB. sesame seeds, for garnish

1. Combine soy sauce, olive oil, sesame oil, and molasses, and mix well in a blender.

2. Combine spinach, water chestnuts, bean sprouts, and eggs in a serving bowl; toss with dressing and serve. Garnish with slivered almonds and sesame seeds.

RECIPE FOR SUCCESS

This salad is just the treat for those who love hot-and-sour soup. The sweet and spicy flavors in the dressing make this salad irresistible; add seafood or meat for a wonderful main dish salad.

Caesar Salad

Yield:	Serving size:	Prep time:	Cook time:
6 servings	1 cup	10 minutes	1 minute
Each serving has:			
2 g carbohydrate	1 g fiber	3 g protein	

1 large egg

1 tsp. Dijon mustard

2 TB. lemon juice

$\frac{1}{2}$ tsp. salt

1 tsp. freshly ground black pepper

1 clove garlic, minced, or 1 tsp. garlic powder

3 TB. olive oil

1 tsp. anchovy paste

2 heads (6 cups) romaine lettuce, washed and torn into bite-size pieces

2 TB. grated Parmesan cheese

1. Boil egg for 1 minute, remove shell, and set aside. In a small bowl, combine mustard, lemon juice, salt, pepper, and garlic; whisk together until salt dissolves.

2. Add oil, anchovy paste, and boiled egg and mix until well blended. Toss with romaine lettuce; sprinkle with Parmesan and serve.

RECIPE FOR SUCCESS

Most Caesar salads are served garnished with high-carb croutons. For an extra crunch, try broken pieces of Parmesan crackers or sprinkle with sesame seeds or your favorite nut.

Retro Asparagus Salad

Yield:	Serving size:	Prep time:	Cook time:
6 servings	1 piece	20 minutes plus overnight chill time	5 minutes

Each serving has:			
3 g carbohydrate	3 g fiber	13 g protein	

2 pkg. unflavored gelatin	¾ cup celery, thinly sliced
1¾ cups warm water	2 TB. lemon juice
¼ cup white vinegar	1 (4-oz.) jar pimientos, chopped
2 (10.5-oz.) cans whole asparagus spears, drained well, 1 cup juice reserved	½ cup pecans or walnuts, chopped

1. Dissolve gelatin in ¾ cup water. Boil vinegar with remaining 1 cup water and 1 cup asparagus juice, adding additional water if needed to make 2 cups. Cool slightly.

2. Line an 8-inch-square glass baking dish with drained asparagus spears. Mix gelatin mixture with celery, lemon juice, pimientos, and pecans, and pour over asparagus. Chill overnight to set. Cut into 6 pieces, and serve each on lettuce leaf.

RECIPE FOR SUCCESS

This makes a pretty salad to serve. It is so light it goes well with most meats and casseroles. You can substitute long whole green beans if desired. With the red pimientos, this salad goes well with red and green holiday decorations!

Mandarin Orange Spinach

Yield:	Serving size:	Prep time:	Cook time:
6 servings	1½ cups	15 minutes	None

Each serving has:		
11 g carbohydrate	4 g fiber	7 g protein

1 head romaine lettuce leaves

2 bunches spinach or other greens

3 green onions, sliced

½ bunch fresh parsley, chopped

1 (6-oz.) can Mandarin oranges, drained

4 oz. cashews

¼ cup olive oil

2 TB. wine vinegar

½ tsp. salt

1 tsp. hot sauce (optional)

Freshly ground black pepper to taste

1. Mix together lettuce, spinach, green onions, parsley, oranges, and cashews in a large bowl.

2. In a screw-top jar, mix together oil, vinegar, salt, hot sauce (if using), and pepper; shake well. Pour over salad and serve.

RECIPE FOR SUCCESS

This sweet-hot dressing is delicious served over any greens. Add chunky chicken for a wonderful main dish salad. Or add other fruits such as apples or strawberries.

Marinated Tomato Slices with Mozzarella

Yield:	Serving size:	Prep time:	Cook time:
6 servings	$\frac{1}{6}$ recipe or 4 slices	10 minutes plus 4 hours marinating time	None

Each serving has:			
4 g carbohydrate	2 g fiber	8 g protein	

$\frac{1}{2}$ cup balsamic vinegar

$\frac{1}{2}$ cup olive oil

Salt and freshly ground black pepper to taste

3 TB. fresh basil

6 firm tomatoes, each sliced into 4 to 5 slices

6 slices mozzarella cheese, cut in strips

1. Mix vinegar, oil, salt, pepper, and basil until well combined. Place tomato slices in single layer, and pour marinade over all.

2. Cover and refrigerate at least 4 hours or overnight. Serve on lettuce leaf. Place mozzarella on tomatoes.

RECIPE FOR SUCCESS

This is a wonderful marinade to use especially for fresh tomatoes right from the garden. Add blanched carrots or cucumbers and green beans for a delightful fresh vegetable salad. Marinated tomatoes give a pungent bite to a grilled burger as well.

Marinated Vegetables

Yield:	Serving size:	Prep time:	Cook time:
6 servings	$\frac{3}{4}$ cup or $\frac{1}{6}$ recipe	20 minutes plus overnight chill time	3 minutes

Each serving has:			
3 g carbohydrate	2 g fiber	1 g protein	

1 cup carrot sticks, sliced

1 cup yellow squash, peeled and cubed

1 head fresh broccoli, cut off ends and slice into spears

$1\frac{1}{2}$ cups red wine vinegar

2 TB. water

$\frac{1}{2}$ cup olive oil

1 tsp. brown sugar

1 tsp. spicy mustard

1 tsp. Worcestershire sauce

1 TB. dill seed

$\frac{1}{2}$ tsp. garlic, minced

Salt and freshly ground black pepper to taste

1. Blanch carrot sticks in boiling water for 3 minutes; remove and drain. In a large bowl, mix carrots with squash and broccoli. (If desired, trim broccoli stalks and peel off outer tough portion; slice inner hearts into thin, bite-size pieces.)

2. Mix together vinegar, water, oil, brown sugar, mustard, Worcestershire sauce, dill seed, garlic, salt, and pepper. Pour marinade over vegetables, cover, and chill overnight.

Variation: To make a warm marinated vegetable dish, try using halved, steamed brussels sprouts. Heat marinade until just simmering, pour marinade over warm brussels sprouts, add sliced green onions, mix well, and serve. If desired, refrigerate the dish overnight and serve cold.

RECIPE FOR SUCCESS

You can also marinate blanched green beans or cauliflower, fresh mushrooms, jicama, and so on. It is convenient if you keep a large jar of marinade in the refrigerator; just add extra cut vegetables to the jar as you use them for other dishes. As you make another dish, you can slice an additional onion or bell pepper to add to the marinating vegetables. This vegetable mix makes tasty additions to your green salad.

Mushroom-Artichoke Salad

Yield:	Serving size:	Prep time:	Cook time:
6 servings	⅙ recipe or ½ cup	15 minutes plus overnight chill time	1 minute

Each serving has:			
10 g carbohydrate	9 g fiber	7 g protein	

1 lb. fresh mushrooms, sliced

1 (4-oz.) jar green pitted olives, sliced

1 (3.8-oz.) can black pitted olives, sliced

2 (14-oz.) cans artichoke hearts, cut in quarters

For salad dressing:

1 TB. pimiento, chopped

1 tsp. garlic, minced

½ cup olive oil

½ cup red wine vinegar

½ tsp. dried tarragon, oregano, or dill

Salt and freshly ground black pepper to taste

1. Sauté mushrooms 1 minute and drain. Drain green and black olives, and mix together with artichoke hearts and mushrooms.

2. Combine pimiento, garlic, oil, vinegar, tarragon, salt, and pepper. Pour dressing over vegetables and refrigerate overnight.

Ranch Dressing

Yield:	Serving size:	Prep time:	Cook time:
1½ cups	2 tablespoons	10 minutes	None

Each serving has:			
1 g carbohydrate	0 g fiber	< 1 g protein	

1 cup mayonnaise

¼ cup plain yogurt

¼ cup heavy cream

1 TB. garlic, minced

2 TB. onion, minced

½ tsp. freshly ground black pepper

1. Combine mayonnaise, yogurt, cream, garlic, onion, and pepper until mixed well. Refrigerate to store. Will keep 3 months.

Buttermilk Herb Dressing

Yield:	Serving size:	Prep time:	Cook time:
1 cup	2 tablespoons	10 minutes	None

Each serving has:		
3 g carbohydrate	0 g fiber	1 g protein

¾ cup buttermilk

¼ cup mayonnaise

1 tsp. white pepper

2 tsp. fresh basil, minced or 1 tsp. dried

2 tsp. fresh parsley, minced or ½ tsp. dried

2 cloves garlic, minced

1. Combine buttermilk, mayonnaise, pepper, basil, parsley, and garlic until mixed well. Refrigerate to store. Will keep 3 months.

Dijon-Lemon Vinaigrette

Yield:	Serving size:	Prep time:	Cook time:
¾ cup	2 tablespoons	10 minutes	None

Each serving has:		
1 g carbohydrate	0 g fiber	1 g protein

¼ cup chicken broth or water

3 TB. lemon juice

3 TB. olive oil

3 TB. red wine vinegar

1 TB. Dijon mustard

2 cloves garlic, minced

1 TB. Worcestershire sauce

2 tsp. white pepper

1. Combine broth, lemon juice, olive oil, vinegar, mustard, garlic, Worcestershire sauce, and pepper until mixed well. Refrigerate to store. Will keep for 6 months.

Green Goddess Dressing

Yield:	Serving size:	Prep time:	Cook time:
4½ cups	2 tablespoons	10 minutes	None

Each serving has:			
2 g carbohydrate	0 g fiber	1 g protein	

1 cup sour cream

1 cup mayonnaise

2½ cups whipping cream

3 green onion tops, chopped

2 cloves garlic, minced

1 TB. anchovy paste

1 tsp. white pepper

2 tsp. fresh parsley, minced or
½ tsp. dried

1. Combine sour cream, mayonnaise, whipping cream, green onions, garlic, anchovy paste, pepper, and parsley until mixed well. Refrigerate to store. Will keep 3 months.

RECIPE FOR SUCCESS

Nothing beats the taste of fresh homemade salad dressings. Perk them up with your own favorite seasonings and a variety of flavored vinegars. You know you can pronounce the name of your ingredients with no hidden harmful fats or chemicals.

The Least You Need to Know

- Side salads make an easy, quick, and low-carb way to add texture, fiber, interest, and nutrients to a meal.
- Make dressings from cold expeller-pressed oils for taste and health.
- Add pizzazz to salads with interesting ingredients such as nuts, croutons, pieces of meat or fish, and cheese.
- Eat salads anytime—even for breakfast.

Chapter 21

Fruit Side Dishes

In This Chapter

- Adding fruit to your eating plan
- Sweetening meals with fruit
- Fitting fruit into your carb allotment
- Enjoying fruit's flavors and textures

Fruits are such an important part of a nutritionally sound eating plan that we've given them an entire chapter. Fruits are delicious, satisfying, and convenient. Many fruits, such as oranges, bananas, avocados, and apples, even come naturally packaged in a "to-go" wrapper.

Yes, fruits contain carbs, but they also contain lots of vitamins, minerals, antioxidants, and dietary fiber that are wonderful for your overall health. Perhaps you have avoided eating fruits because you thought they were too high in carbs. They're not as bad as you think. Let's do a quick calculation. One half an apple, which is considered a serving, only has 11 grams carbs and 2.5 grams dietary fiber, for a net carbohydrate value of only 8.5 carbs. Your overall eating plan can easily accommodate an apple; yes, even an apple a day.

Dietitians and nutritionists recommend we eat a minimum of 5 servings of fruits and vegetables a day. They know the importance of fruits to your health and well-being. Plus, there are tastes and textures in fruits that you just can't get anywhere else. They'll add wonderful variety and interest to your meals. In other words, it's time to start enjoying fruit.

Dessert or Side Dish

Eating fruits is an excellent way to satisfy your sweet tooth. The fructose, or fruit sugar, in fruits makes them sweet. Fructose is low glycemic, meaning that it causes only a small rise in blood sugar levels when eaten in its natural form in whole fruit, which is good. So you can eat moderate serving sizes of fruit and satisfy your sweet tooth while eating low glycemic, which is good for your heart, your weight, and your health.

Fruits are a versatile food eaten in several ways: as a snack, a side dish, or as a dessert. You can serve these recipes as side dishes for breakfast, lunch, or dinner. You can also serve them as desserts or snacks. You get to choose how fruit works in your eating plans.

Nutritionists now recommend we "eat a rainbow." In other words, eat many colors of foods daily. Eat foods that are green, yellow, purple, red, orange, and even blue. Like vegetables, fruits have many varied colors. Both provide unique nutrients that help strengthen the immune system, protect against free radical damage, help prevent cancer, and in short, keep our bodies functioning well.

HOT POTATO

Some fruit, such as bananas, pineapple, papaya, watermelon, and apricots, are moderate glycemic. Eat them in moderate amounts. You'll get the pleasure and nutrition they offer without straying from your eating plan.

Into Your Meal

These fruit recipes have been designed to be low carb. We have taken advantage of the natural sweetness of fruit to save you carbs while letting you enjoy the benefits that cooking with fruit provides. The fruit in these recipes are mostly used raw but are sometimes cooked. Either way, they provide similar nutritional value.

If you are carefully counting carbohydrate grams, find a way to add at least 1 fruit a day. If you are more relaxed about your carb counts, then eat more.

Fresh Fruit Medley with Poppy Seed Dressing

Yield:	Serving size:	Prep time:	Cook time:
8 servings	$\frac{1}{8}$ recipe	25 minutes	None

Each serving has:			
14 g carbohydrate	3 g fiber	1 g protein	

1 orange, peeled and cut into sections

1 grapefruit, peeled and cut into bite-size sections

1 banana, peeled and sliced

1 apple (Fuji, JonaGold, or Pink Lady), cored and sliced

1 pint strawberries, stemmed and cut in half

1 pear, cored and cut into 1-in. pieces

5 sprigs fresh basil, cut into 1-in. pieces

3 TB. fresh or bottled lemon juice, divided

$\frac{1}{4}$ cup walnut oil, cold expeller-pressed

$1\frac{1}{2}$ tsp. poppy seeds

1 tsp. honey

Salt and freshly ground black pepper to taste

1. Combine orange, grapefruit, banana, apple, strawberries, and pear in a large bowl with basil. Toss with 1 tablespoon lemon juice to keep fruits from discoloring.

2. Make dressing by combining walnut oil, remaining 2 tablespoons lemon juice, poppy seeds, honey, and salt and pepper to taste. Pour dressing over fruit mixture, and toss to coat fruits. Serve immediately.

Variation: Make this recipe with whatever fresh fruit is available locally in your grocery store. You can also add chopped or slivered nuts, such as pecans, pine nuts, walnuts, almonds, macadamias, and pistachios. Or add seeds—pumpkin, flax, sesame, or sunflower.

TABLE TALK

Cold expeller-pressed means the oil was pressed out of the walnuts rather than using heat. When vegetable and nut oils are heated, which is more common, they change into trans-fatty acids, which directly cause heart disease.

Apples with Raisins and Pecans

Yield:	Serving size:	Prep time:	Cook time:
8 servings	⅛ recipe	25 minutes	25 minutes

Each serving has:		
14 g carbohydrate	3 g fiber	1 g protein

4 medium apples, cored and sliced (your favorite)	2 TB. fresh or bottled lemon juice
½ tsp. cinnamon	¼ cup raisins
½ tsp. nutmeg	½ cup pecan halves
	2 TB. butter

1. Preheat the oven to 350°F.

2. Put apples, cinnamon, nutmeg, lemon juice, and raisins into a baking dish and mix. Spread evenly with pecans and dot with small pieces of butter. Bake, covered, for 25 minutes.

RECIPE FOR SUCCESS

We used a favorite pie recipe and took away the crust. We think you'll love the filling as much as we do. It's a terrific combination of tastes. Use this recipe as a dessert or as a side dish with eggs for breakfast.

Gingered Papayas

Yield:	Serving size:	Prep time:	Cook time:
8 servings	½ papaya	10 minutes	30 minutes

Each serving has:		
12 g carbohydrate	3 g fiber	1 g protein

4 firm, ripe papayas, halved and hollowed	1 tsp. ground ginger
8 TB. butter (1 stick)	8 thin slices lime
4 TB. fresh or bottled lime juice	Dash cayenne

1. Preheat the oven to 350°F.

2. Cut papayas in half lengthwise, and scoop out seeds. Arrange in a glass baking dish with ¹⁄₈ inch warm water in the bottom. In each papaya hollow, place 1 tablespoon butter, ¹⁄₂ tablespoon lime juice, and ¹⁄₈ teaspoon ground ginger.

3. Bake for 30 minutes, basting 10 minutes before done. Place a slice of lime at the edge of each papaya half. Add a dash cayenne and serve warm.

RECIPE FOR SUCCESS

Papayas bring the taste of the tropics into our kitchens. Baking them brings out their flavor, which also is enhanced by the butter. To ripen fruit, place in a closed container, such as a paper bag. Fruit gives off ethylene gas, which hastens the ripening process. A closed container concentrates the gas, and the fruit ripens more quickly. Serve as a dessert or side dish for brunch.

Fresh Berries with Orange Cream

Yield:	Serving size:	Prep time:	Cook time:
4 servings	¹⁄₄ recipe	15 minutes	15 minutes
Each serving has:			
12 g carbohydrate	2 g fiber	2 g protein	

1 pint strawberries, washed, hulled, and sliced in half (leaving whole is optional)

1 TB. sugar

2 tsp. orange zest, grated

¹⁄₂ cup orange juice

1 cup heavy cream

1. Combine sugar, orange zest, and orange juice in a small saucepan. Bring to a boil, stirring only until sugar dissolves. Simmer 10 minutes without stirring. Cool completely.

2. Whip cream until soft peaks form. Gently fold in orange syrup. Serve over berries.

Variation: Substitute fresh blueberries or raspberries, and, instead of orange, use lemon juice and rind in the same quantities.

RECIPE FOR SUCCESS

This recipe makes a great side dish for a meat entrée, or serve it as dessert.

Waldorf Salad

Yield:	Serving size:	Prep time:	Cook time:
6 servings	¾ cup	20 minutes	None

Each serving has:		
4 g carbohydrate	2 g fiber	3 g protein

1 cup celery, diced	½ cup walnuts or pecans, chopped
1 cup apples, diced	¾ cup mayonnaise
1 cup green grapes, halved	

1. Combine celery, apples, grapes, walnuts, and mayonnaise. Mix well.

RECIPE FOR SUCCESS

This crunchy, sweet, and at the same time tangy combination of ingredients goes well with virtually all main dishes. The fruits are available year-round at the grocery store, so you can serve this for Thanksgiving dinner or a summer barbecue. But remember, as this dish is mayonnaise-based, keep it refrigerated until serving and don't keep it out in the hot sun, as it will turn bad.

Avocado and Papaya Salad

Yield:	Serving size:	Prep time:	Cook time:
6 servings	⅙ recipe	20 minutes	None

Each serving has:		
4 g carbohydrate	3 g fiber	1 g protein

1 cup avocado, cubed	1 TB. lime juice
1 papaya, peeled and sliced diagonally	¼ tsp. paprika
6 Bibb lettuce leaves	½ tsp. salt
For dressing:	½ tsp. dry mustard
½ cup olive oil	1 tsp. onion, minced
⅓ cup tarragon vinegar	1½ TB. papaya seeds

1. Arrange avocado and papaya on a lettuce leaf.

2. To make dressing, place oil, vinegar, lime juice, paprika, salt, mustard, and onion into a blender. Cover and blend thoroughly. Add papaya seeds and blend until seeds are the size of coarsely ground pepper. Chill.

3. Pour dressing over fruit just before serving.

RECIPE FOR SUCCESS

Enjoy this wonderful fruit salad with your meals. You get an extra bonus if you serve it with a hearty meat main course. The ground-up papaya seeds in the dressing plus the papaya itself offer a high amount of natural digestive enzymes.

TABLE TALK

Papaya seeds are edible. Most people only eat the sweet delicious flesh, but you can also eat the small, black seeds in the center of the fruit. The seeds taste like black pepper and contain papain, a digestive enzyme. The ground seeds can also be used in marinades to tenderize meat. People in some countries use papaya seeds in place of black peppercorns.

Pears with Avocado and Lime

Yield:	Serving size:	Prep time:	Cook time:
6 servings	$\frac{1}{6}$ recipe	20 minutes	None
Each serving has:			
14 g carbohydrate	6 g fiber	1 g protein	

2 TB. water

2 tsp. lime zest, finely grated

$\frac{1}{4}$ cup fresh lime juice

3 firm, ripe pears, peeled and sliced

$1\frac{1}{2}$ cups avocado, halved, pitted, removed from skin, and sliced

1 head red leaf lettuce, leaves left whole

$\frac{1}{4}$ cup fresh cilantro, chopped

1. Into water, stir lime zest and lime juice and set aside. Brush pear and each avocado slice with lime juice mixture to prevent discoloration.

2. Arrange lettuce leaves on individual serving plates. Alternate slices of pear and avocado over lettuce. Top with additional lime juice mixture and sprinkle with cilantro.

RECIPE FOR SUCCESS

Enjoy avocado any way you can. It is filled with good and healthy fats and offers high nutritional value. It's great with lime, but it's fabulous with pears and lime.

Fruit Salad with Passion Fruit

Yield:	Serving size:	Prep time:	Cook time:
6 servings	2 cups	20 minutes plus chill time	None

Each serving has:		
9 g carbohydrate	3 g fiber	< 1 g protein

2 cups strawberries, hulled and halved

2 oranges, peeled and segmented

2 passion fruit, halved

3 TB. walnut oil

2 TB. white wine

¼ tsp. ginger

1. Put strawberries and oranges into a serving bowl. Using a teaspoon, scoop flesh of passion fruit into the bowl.

2. Mix walnut oil, white wine, and ginger in a small bowl. Pour mixture over fruit and toss gently. Cover and chill in the refrigerator until ready to serve.

Variation: You can substitute grapefruit for the oranges and raspberries for the strawberries in this recipe. Also, instead of passion fruit, you can use pomegranate seeds. For a special taste, substitute 1 teaspoon poppy seeds for the ginger.

Pear Compote

Yield:	Serving size:	Prep time:	Cook time:
6 servings	1 pear plus $\frac{1}{6}$ sauce	10 minutes	20 to 30 minutes

Each serving has:		
20 g carbohydrate	5 g fiber	1 g protein

6 firm pears, peeled, cores removed, and halved

2 cups boiling water

$\frac{1}{4}$ tsp. fresh ginger, minced

1 slice lemon

2 TB. pistachios, chopped

1. Drop pears into boiling water, cover, and simmer 10 minutes.

2. Add ginger and lemon. Cover and cook until tender, about 10 to 20 minutes. To serve, sprinkle with pistachios.

RECIPE FOR SUCCESS

Pears are great eaten fresh or cooked. Poached pears make a great treat, and this recipe is low carb. Serve with a slice of lemon and garnish with mint.

Curried Fruit on Skewers

Yield:	Serving size:	Prep time:	Cook time:
8 servings	1 skewer	20 minutes plus overnight chill time	1 hour

Each serving has:		
18 g carbohydrate	3 g fiber	1 g protein

1 (8-oz.) can unsweetened pineapple rings

1 (16-oz.) can unsweetened pear halves

1 (16-oz.) can unsweetened peach halves

8 green grapes

$\frac{1}{2}$ cup butter (1 stick)

1 TB. molasses

1 TB. curry powder

1. Soak 8 bamboo skewers in water for 30 minutes.

2. Preheat the oven to 350°F.

3. Drain pineapple, pears, and peaches, and pat dry with paper towels. Make fruit skewers with 8 bamboo skewers by placing 1 pineapple ring on the bottom, top with pear half, then peach half, and then green grape. Secure stacks with toothpicks, and place in a shallow baking dish.

4. In a small saucepan, melt butter. Stir in molasses and curry powder. Spoon mixture over fruit, and bake covered for 1 hour. Refrigerate overnight before serving.

RECIPE FOR SUCCESS

The flavors in this recipe continue to blend for several days. You can use less curry powder if you prefer a lighter taste. Garnish with fresh basil or mint leaves.

Frosty Fruit

Yield:	Serving size:	Prep time:	Cook time:
6 servings	¾ cup	15 minutes plus overnight freezing time	None

Each serving has:		
13 g carbohydrate	4 g fiber	4 g protein

1 (8-oz.) can pineapple pieces packed in water

½ cup walnut halves

2 TB. lime juice

¼ tsp. ground ginger

3 cups fresh or frozen strawberry halves, no added sugar

1½ cups fresh or frozen blueberries, no added sugar

¼ cup unsweetened coconut

1. Combine undrained pineapple tidbits, walnut halves, lime juice, and ginger. Mix well and add strawberries, blueberries, and coconut. Toss gently.

2. Freeze overnight. Thaw about 4 hours, and serve while frosty.

RECIPE FOR SUCCESS

This fruit combination makes a great addition to lunchboxes. Freeze in individual containers and add to the lunchbox in the morning. By lunch time, the fruit should be partly thawed and frosty.

Microwave Cheesy Apples

Yield:	Serving size:	Prep time:	Cook time:
1 serving	1 apple	5 minutes	4 minutes

Each serving has:		
21 g carbohydrate	4 g fiber	7 g protein

1 medium cooking apple (such as Gala, Macintosh, Golden Delicious, or Cortland), cored, peeled (optional), and quartered

¼ to ½ tsp. cinnamon

¼ cup cheddar cheese, shredded

1. Core apple and cut into quarters. Peel it, if desired. Place apple on microwave-safe plate, and sprinkle with cinnamon. Microwave on high for 3 minutes.

2. Sprinkle with cheese, and microwave 1 minute. Let cool slightly before serving.

RECIPE FOR SUCCESS

This recipe is a perfect snack, as it includes fiber as well as protein and no added sugar but will fill the need for healthy carbs. Try this snack with a fresh pear and Swiss cheese for a new flavor. The kids will love this quick and easy after-school snack, or serve it up for a warm breakfast to get them going—and you, too!

Minty Fruit

Yield:	Serving size:	Prep time:	Cook time:
6 servings	¾ cup	15 minutes plus chill time	None

Each serving has:		
12 g carbohydrate	2 g fiber	1 g protein

2 TB. mayonnaise

1 TB. fresh or bottled lemon juice

2 TB. cream cheese, softened

2 tsp. fresh mint or ½ tsp. dried

2 cups fresh strawberries, cut in half

1 cup fresh or frozen blueberries, no added sugar

1 banana, cut into chunks

1 cup cantaloupe, cubed or honeydew melon or a mixture

1. In a small container, combine mayonnaise, sugar, lemon juice, cream cheese, and mint.

2. Lightly toss together strawberries, blueberries, banana, and cantaloupe, and stir in mayonnaise dressing. Chill before serving.

RECIPE FOR SUCCESS

This is a pretty dish to serve in parfait glasses with a fresh strawberry wedged on the rim of the glass. It makes a refreshing dessert or snack and is a great way to add fruit to breakfast.

The Least You Need to Know

- Eating fruits is a wise choice for nutritional value and mealtime variety.
- Most fruits are low glycemic, but some fruits fall into the moderate-glycemic range.
- Eat fruits any time of the day for snacks, side dishes, or desserts.
- Before you make fruit purchases, consider the way you are going to use the fruit.

Extras: Treats and Starches

The extras are those foods you may think are forbidden in low-carb eating. They aren't forbidden here, just reformulated with low-carb ingredients that taste decadently rich!

You'll love the chocolate brownies, the peach ice cream, and the walnut torte. If bread is your passion, make up a batch of Rice Flour Rolls or Almond Crackers.

These recipes will delight you with their high-carb tastes that fit into your low-carb daily allotments.

Breads and Pasta

In This Chapter

- Enjoying breads
- Low-carb bread ingredients
- Preparation hints
- Slicing it thin

Bread has been called the staff of life. Perhaps that no longer rings true for you. Your new staff of life might be a balanced combination of vegetables, fruits, and protein. Does that mean that bread with its hefty dose of carbs doesn't have a place in your life? You'll probably be eating it very sparingly and likely a new type of bread. It will be of the whole-grain and low-carb varieties.

Your new bread is made with ingredients that can be filling but not high in carbohydrates. Out goes the refined wheat flour; in go such ingredients as nut flours, psyllium, oat bran, and soy powder. You can enjoy low-carb bread in slices or rolls for such foods as hamburgers and hot dogs. You can eat low-carb crackers with cheese or nut butters. And you can make scrumptious croutons for your salads.

Eating Bread

Low-carb bread almost by definition doesn't contain much, if any, high-carbohydrate flours. All grain-based highly refined flours such as whole wheat, white, and rye contain way too many carbohydrates for you—that is, if the breads are made the regular way. One possible way for you to eat regular flour breads is to slice them so thin that you are actually eating only $\frac{1}{3}$ to $\frac{1}{2}$ a serving. Quite honestly, that works. Eating less of any carbohydrate-rich food reduces the amount of carbohydrates you ingest.

Another choice is to eat low-carb bread. Yes, you can purchase low-carb breads at the grocery and health food stores. Some regular wheat breads are labeled "low carb" because they deliver fewer carbohydrates per slice. This is because the bread is sliced ³⁄₈-inch thick rather than the usual ⁵⁄₈ inch. So simply by the baker controlling portion size, the bread has fewer carbohydrates.

Components of Low-Carb Bread

In creating a low-carb version of the "staff of life," let's look at what exactly makes bread become bread. Bread dough requires the following components:

- **Leavening.** This is the ingredient that puts the air holes into the bread. For yeast breads, that ingredient is yeast; in other breads, it's baking powder or baking soda. Flat breads, such as crackers, usually don't contain leavening. Low-carb breads use the same leavening as regular breads.

- **"Stick-together-ness."** To make bread, there has to be an ingredient that makes the ingredient mixture stick together. One of the unique qualities of wheat is that it contains gluten. When kneaded, the gluten develops, and causes the bread mixture to stick together. Low-carb yeast breads often forego the actual high-carb wheat and instead use "vital wheat gluten," available at grocery stores. For flat breads made with nut flours, the stick-together ingredient is eggs.

- **Filling.** This ingredient makes up the greatest volume of the bread. In regular bread, it is flour; in low-carb breads, it could be a combination of bran, psyllium, soy, or whey flours. These contain fewer carbs than wheat flour.

- **Sugar.** Yeast breads need some form of sugar for the yeast to feed upon and, thus, to grow. This can be a very small amount of sugar, honey, or molasses and these are called for in some of our yeast low-carb breads.

You can bake your own bread with the recipes in this chapter. We offer you yeast breads and quick breads, so you can make the kind you prefer. Plus, you can enjoy the warm satisfaction that comes from both the baking and the eating. There's nothing like fresh-out-of-the-oven bread to warm the heart and home.

TABLE TALK

Brushing breads with a glaze or egg wash before baking gives the final product a brown patina and crisp finish. The most basic wash is water, which gives the crust a little shine. Milk brushed on a loaf of bread gives a luster to the normally matte finish. Whole eggs beaten with a pinch of salt give an even golden finish; egg white alone gets glossy, and crusts brushed with yolks become almost burnished.

"Special" Ingredients

These recipes call for some special ingredients, which you can find at large grocery stores, health food stores, or via mail order online.

- **Vital wheat gluten.** This is the protein component of wheat that makes all the ingredients stick together. By using only the gluten from the wheat and not the wheat itself, you reduce the carbohydrate count.

- **Psyllium husk.** Psyllium contains a water-soluble fiber that has been used for thousands of years for stomach and digestive health. It has no net carbohydrates but adds plenty of good-for-you fiber to the bread.

- **Nut flours.** You can purchase these or make them yourself. To make 1 cup nut flour, process ¾ cup nuts in the food processor until they turn into a flour. Almonds, pecans, walnuts, macadamias, and hazelnuts all work well.

- **Soy powder or soy milk powder.** Soy powder or soy milk powder is made from cooked soybeans and adds a nutritional filler and wheat flour substitute for bread. Do not use soy flour, as it has a stronger taste. And don't use soy protein isolate, either; it is not the same thing. If your health food store doesn't stock soy powder, have them order it for you.

- **Whey protein powder.** Purchase this without added sugar. The plain, unsweetened version works well as an ingredient in low-carb breads, plus it adds more protein to the bread.

- **Rice flour.** This is a great ingredient for bread. We use this in some recipes to offer you another choice of grain if you are sensitive to wheat.

- **Oat bran.** As the outer husk of oats, the bran has lots of good-for-you water-soluble fiber.

Keep these staple ingredients in stock in your pantry just as you would wheat flour, so they'll be there when you want to make some low-carb bread.

TABLE TALK

For spaghetti or fettuccine, we prefer using spaghetti squash. One of Lucy's favorite recipes is Spaghetti Squash with Marinara Sauce in Chapter 19.

Pastas

Some low-carb pastas are commercially available in stores. You can try some and determine if you like them. Typically they are either too stiff or too pasty. But new brands are coming out continually, and hopefully, you'll find one that appeals to you.

We have found that using vegetables in place of pasta is delicious and quite satisfying. Try using zucchini in lasagna. You can also use other vegetables such as bamboo shoots, turnips, fennel, beets, carrots, broccoli, and cauliflower in place of wheat pasta.

Vegetables as pasta give you a lighter feeling after eating, and, of course, they add 1 or even 2 more vegetables to your daily fruits and vegetables target of 5 to 10 each day. To tell you the truth, we prefer vegetables to wheat- and rice-based pasta.

Cheese Bread

Yield:	Serving size:	Prep time:	Cook time:
16 servings	1 slice	10 minutes	45 minutes
Each serving has:			
1 g carbohydrate	0 g fiber	14 g protein	

²⁄₃ cup soy powder

²⁄₃ cup whey protein powder

1 tsp. baking powder

4 large eggs

2 TB. sour cream

2 TB. butter

1 tsp. basil or rosemary

2 cups cheddar cheese (or any type you prefer), shredded

1. Preheat the oven to 275°F.

2. Combine soy powder, whey protein powder, baking powder, eggs, sour cream, butter, basil, and cheddar cheese, and pour into greased 4 × 8 × 4-inch loaf pan. Bake 40 minutes. Test with knife for doneness. Cover with aluminum foil if browning too rapidly.

3. Cool loaf completely before slicing into 16 (¹⁄₂-inch) pieces.

Variation: To make Asiago cheese bread, substitute shredded Asiago for the cheddar cheese. To make a sun-dried tomato bread, add 2 tablespoons finely chopped sun-dried tomatoes.

RECIPE FOR SUCCESS

The thinner the slices, the better the flavor and texture. Toasting brings out the best flavor. Instead of using herbs, substitute ¼ cup chopped olives. For a sweeter-tasting bread, use almond flavoring with no herbs or olives and only 1 cup of a mild-flavored cheese.

Rice Flour Rolls

Yield:	Serving size:	Prep time:	Cook time:
12 servings	1 roll	10 minutes	20 minutes

Each serving has:		
5 g carbohydrate	0 g fiber	10 g protein

3 TB. rice flour	6 TB. butter
¾ cup vital wheat gluten	2 large eggs
¼ tsp. salt	3 egg whites
1 cup minus 2 TB. heavy cream	

1. Preheat the oven to 425°F.

2. Combine rice flour, wheat gluten, and salt and set aside. Combine cream and butter in a saucepan, and simmer until butter melts. Remove the pan from heat. Add dry ingredients, and stir quickly until mixed well and dough leaves the sides of the pan.

3. Stir in each egg separately until well combined. Combine all egg whites together with a fork, and add to mixture, stirring well. Pour into 12 greased muffin cups, and bake 20 minutes until golden brown.

Everyday Rolls

Yield:	Serving size:	Prep time:	Cook time:
12 servings	1 roll	10 minutes	12 minutes after rising

Each serving has:		
6 g carbohydrate	2 g fiber	5 g protein

½ cup heavy cream
½ cup water
2 TB. psyllium husks
¾ cup vital wheat gluten
⅓ cup oat bran
½ cup whey protein powder

¼ cup rice flour
1 tsp. salt
1 tsp. vanilla or almond extract
1 TB. melted butter
1 TB. sugar
1 packet rapid-rise yeast

If you're using a bread machine:

1. Place cream, water, psyllium husks, wheat gluten, oat bran, whey protein pow-der, rice flour, salt, vanilla, butter, sugar, and yeast into bread machine in that order, and set the machine for rising only. Remove dough from the pan and pull apart. Either place on a greased baking sheet and shape into rolls, or place in 12 greased muffin tins.

If you're using a conventional oven:

1. Let dough rise covered in draft-free room until doubled in size.

When using bread machine or conventional oven method:

2. Preheat the oven to 375°F.

3. Bake for 12 minutes or until set and a knife inserted into the center of a roll comes out clean.

RECIPE FOR SUCCESS

Shape the rolls into hamburger or hotdog buns if you want to serve with a summer barbecue. You can omit the vanilla or almond flavoring and use vanilla-flavored whey protein powder, if desired.

Variations: Take the dough out of the machine after the first rising, and pat into a rectangle on a greased sheet pan. Sprinkle the dough with your favorite fillings, and roll up jellyroll style. Cover and allow this to rise and then bake in the oven until golden brown. You can do this for any of the yeast breads.

To make a cinnamon roll, lightly sprinkle the dough with cinnamon and a few nuts and raisins; if desired, mix a bit of reduced-carb jelly into the filling. Serve hot with the Pancake Syrup in Chapter 5. You can also layer cooked meats, chopped vegetables, and cheese onto the dough and bake.

Yeast Bread with Seeds

Yield:	Serving size:	Prep time:	Cook time:
12 servings	1 slice	10 minutes	Approx. 3 hours in bread machine

Each serving has:			
6 g carbohydrate	4 g fiber	10 g protein	

1 cup heavy cream
1 TB. melted butter
1 egg, beaten
$\frac{1}{2}$ tsp. salt
2 TB. psyllium husks
$\frac{3}{4}$ cup vital wheat gluten
$\frac{1}{2}$ cup oat bran
$\frac{1}{3}$ cup almond flour ($\frac{1}{4}$ cup almonds, finely ground)

$\frac{1}{4}$ cup sunflower seeds, coarsely chopped
3 TB. whole flax seeds
1 TB. sugar
1 tsp. molasses
1 packet rapid-rise yeast

If you're using a bread machine:

1. Place cream, melted butter, egg, salt, psyllium husks, wheat gluten, oat bran, almond flour, sunflower seeds, flax seeds, sugar, molasses, and yeast into a bread machine in that order and bake. Remove bread from the pan immediately, and allow to cool before slicing into 12 servings.

If you're using a conventional oven:

1. Preheat the oven to 350°F.

2. Combine liquid ingredients. In a separate bowl, combine dry ingredients with yeast.

3. Make a hole in the center of dry ingredients, and pour in liquid ingredients. Slowly stir to combine completely.

4. Pour into a greased 4 × 8 × 4-inch loaf pan or 2 smaller pans. Bake 25 to 30 minutes. Test with a knife for doneness. Cover with some aluminum foil if bread is browning too rapidly.

Variation: You can use many different kinds of seeds or nuts in this bread. Choose from pumpkin seeds, pine nuts, sesame seeds, pecans, walnuts, and even poppy seeds.

 RECIPE FOR SUCCESS

Toasting this bread makes the nutty flavor come alive. Add a slice of cheese and melt for a quick and nutritious breakfast.

Chewy Low-Carb Bread

Yield:	Serving size:	Prep time:	Cook time:
10 servings	1 slice	10 minutes	3 hours
Each serving has:			
5 g carbohydrate	1 g fiber	14 g protein	

1 TB. olive oil

1/2 cup warm water (95°F–105°F)

1/2 cup cream

1 egg, at room temperature

1 cup plus 2 TB. vital wheat gluten

1/2 cup oat flour

1/2 cup plain whey protein powder

1 tsp. vanilla extract

1/4 tsp. salt

1 package rapid-rise yeast

If you're using a bread machine:

1. Add oil to bottom of a bread machine pan.

2. Use a thermometer to determine the temperature of water; if it is too hot, it will kill yeast. Slightly warm cream, and add to water in a large bowl. Slightly beat egg, and add to cream mixture. Pour into a bread machine pan.

3. In a large bowl, combine gluten, oat flour, whey powder, vanilla, and salt. Mix thoroughly and gently pour onto top of cream mixture, but do not stir into cream mixture. Sprinkle yeast on top of flour mixture.

4. Set the machine to rapid bake setting, which is usually about 2 hours with one knead cycle. Check the manufacturer's directions for your machine. When bread has cooled, slice loaf into 10 slices.

If you're using a conventional oven:

1. Preheat the oven to 350°F.

2. Combine liquid ingredients plus vanilla. In a separate bowl, combine dry ingredients with yeast.

3. Make a hole in the center of the dry ingredients, and pour in liquid ingredients. Slowly stir to combine completely.

4. Pour into greased 4 × 8 × 4-inch loaf pan or 2 smaller pans. Bake 25 to 30 minutes. Test with a knife for doneness. Cover with some aluminum foil if bread is browning too rapidly.

RECIPE FOR SUCCESS

This really is a chewy bread. Because of the texture, it is quite filling. Add your favorite nuts or cheese for variety. Slice the loaf into thinner slices and toast to make it more flavorful.

Vegetable Pasta

Yield:	Serving size:	Prep time:	Cook time:
2 servings	½ cup	10 minutes plus 30 minutes standing time	2 minutes

Each serving has:		
2 g carbohydrate	2 g fiber	1 g protein

3 (6-in.) zucchini, halved crosswise and then into ⅓-in.-thick lengthwise strips

1 tsp. salt

2 tsp. olive oil

½ tsp. fresh or bottled lemon juice

½ tsp. freshly ground black pepper

1. Cut each strip into ½-inch-thick pieces. Place in a colander, and sprinkle with salt. Let stand for 30 minutes. Rinse and pat dry.

2. Toss in oil, lemon juice, and pepper, and microwave 1 to 2 minutes until tender-crisp. Serve as is or use as "pasta" base for delicious sauces.

Variation: You can also use a vegetable peeler to make "pasta" from other vegetables such as bamboo shoots, turnip, fennel, beet, carrot, and broccoli. These vegetables will not need to be salted and set aside for ½ hour, as they have a high water content like zucchini. First, peel any vegetable with a tough covering; slice thin strips and microwave about 2 minutes just until tender-crisp. Cover with your favorite sauce. Using several vegetables mixed together gives the sauce a wonderful flavor and adds multiple nutrients to your meal.

RECIPE FOR SUCCESS

This recipe is an excellent base for serving with Italian sauces. It takes well to a sprinkling of Italian herbs when tossing. You can also use a vegetable peeler to slice zucchini into thinner strips—just peel and then rotate zucchini around as you slice off pasta strips.

Almond Crackers

Yield:	Serving size:	Prep time:	Cook time:
6 servings	$\frac{1}{6}$ recipe	10 minutes	10 minutes

Each serving has:		
3 g carbohydrate	3 g fiber	12 g protein

$1\frac{3}{4}$ cups almond flour ($1\frac{1}{2}$ cups almonds, finely ground)

3 TB. vital wheat gluten

$\frac{1}{2}$ tsp. salt

1 egg

1 TB. olive oil

1 TB. water

1. Preheat the oven to 350°F.

2. Blend together almond flour, wheat gluten, and salt and set aside. Slightly beat egg with oil and water. Make a well in the middle of flour mixture, and pour in liquid. Mix well until mixture forms a ball.

3. Lightly grease 2 sheets of waxed paper, and place dough between sheets. Roll as thin as possible.

4. Cut dough into desired shapes and sizes, and place on a baking sheet. Bake for about 10 minutes or until golden brown. Watch carefully as they will burn quickly.

5. Cool and serve. Seal leftovers in a closed container.

Variation: Vary the taste of these crackers by substituting other nut flours. You can use pecans, walnuts, macadamias, pine nuts, and hazelnuts.

RECIPE FOR SUCCESS

These crackers are delicious. Add spices or seasonings as desired to batter before cooking or use garlic salt. The thinner the dough is rolled out, the crisper the cracker will be. These crackers are wonderful with dips and salsa, or use them with cheese for a late-afternoon snack.

Croutons

Yield:	Serving size:	Prep time:	Cook time:
16 servings	2 tablespoons	10 minutes	15 minutes

Each serving has:		
4 g carbohydrate	1 g fiber	1 g protein

4 TB. butter

2 cups cubed day-old bread (preferably French or Asiago cheese bread, but any bread will do)

⅛ tsp. garlic salt

⅛ tsp. dried parsley

Salt and freshly ground black pepper to taste

1. Heat butter in a heavy skillet. Stir in bread cubes, and coat with butter on all sides. Sprinkle on garlic salt, parsley, and salt and pepper to taste. Continue to stir until bread is toasted to your preference.

Variation: Vary the seasonings in this recipe. Use crushed red peppers or hot chili powder. Or use Italian seasonings such as pesto or marinara seasonings.

RECIPE FOR SUCCESS

Croutons are a wonderful way to get small tastes of delicious bread with very few carbohydrates. Be sure to use bread that's been sitting around for several days and is already partially dried out. Sprinkle the croutons on salads, and use the tiniest crumbs to top scrambled eggs. You can also sprinkle them over steamed vegetables.

The Least You Need to Know

- You can enjoy low-carb breads in many forms—sliced, as rolls, muffins, and crackers.
- Baking low-carb breads requires different ingredients than regular high-carb wheat-flour breads.
- Home-baked bread gives you the wonderful satisfaction of the baking, eating, and emotional comforts.
- Vegetable pastas are terrific and so far beat out commercial brands of low-carb pasta.

Grains and Potatoes

In This Chapter

* Enjoying low-carb starches
* Cooking with unrefined whole grains
* Getting that comfort-food taste
* Sticking with serving-size suggestions

Not surprisingly, we have all grown to love grains and potatoes dearly. They appeal to both "mouth and mind." In other words, they taste good and help satisfy our emotional needs as well. We often refer to such starchy foods as "comfort" foods for good reason. A serving of them actually increases serotonin levels in the brain, which make us feel good. We get relaxed and soothed. We might even get sleepy and fall into a deep sleep faster.

Of course, all this happens subconsciously, but it helps explain our devotion to starchy foods. It's part of why many of us return, not just for second helpings of plain-old mashed potatoes but for a third mound of them, too!

When embarking on a low-carb eating regimen, the prospect of never again eating potatoes or rice isn't encouraging. Don't despair. The good news is you can have some starches, as these recipes prove. True, the carb count may be out of range if you are on a highly carb-restricted eating program, but generally speaking, you can eat them once or twice a week and perhaps more often. If you use the mock potato recipes, you can eat them more often.

Choosing Good Grains

For these recipes, we chose whole grains that are low glycemic and unrefined. Unrefined whole grains retain the outer covering of the grain and contain more fiber and more B vitamins than refined grains. Our recipes call for pearl barley, quinoa, and brown basmati rice. Don't be put off by these odd names; they'll easily become family favorites. And they're widely available at regular grocery stores.

But watch out. These grains still contain plenty of carbohydrates, so be sure to eat the recommended serving size to avoid a carb overload. Grains and potatoes go down easily, so don't overdo the quantity consumed. The servings in the recipes here contain around 18 to 22 carbs, so you'll need to make sure your eating plan for the day can "afford" the higher carb counts. You can also eat half the recommended serving size to manage your daily carb allotment and still enjoy the taste of these foods.

We think you'll like the taste of these more unusual grains and find the combination of ingredients delicious. Nuts go well with whole grains, as do fresh parsley, cilantro, dill, and many spices.

> **HOT POTATO**
>
> Rice and potatoes are so easy to eat and so soothing that it's not hard to overeat them. You already know this. The secret to enjoying starches and eating low carb is to eat less. Follow the serving size recommendations carefully, and you'll like the results.

Sweet Potatoes Bring Smiles

With the one exception of the Jalapeño Red Potato Bowls, our potato recipes call for either yams or sweet potatoes. Both have orange-colored insides. Both are lower glycemic than white potatoes but just as delicious.

If you have any reservations about eating yams or sweet potatoes, we challenge you to bake a few. Eat them seasoned with butter, salt, and pepper. You can sprinkle with some cinnamon. You'll be sold on the sweet taste, the texture, and the overall satisfaction you receive. They've become such a staple at our family dinners that our children actually prefer them to white baked potatoes.

Sweet potatoes and yams have about the same carb count as white potatoes, but we recommend them because they're lower glycemic and we think they taste better. Note that the suggested serving is $1/2$ potato.

Ingredients

Barley, quinoa, and brown basmati rice are probably not already in your pantry, as they are less common grains. Here's where to purchase these ingredients and others that we will use in this chapter:

- Brown basmati rice can often be found prepackaged in the rice section, and in bulk bins in the health food section of your grocery store. If not, ask at the health food store. If you still can't find them, search online and purchase in bulk. It stores well and keeps for months in a covered container or plastic bag.

- Pearl barley is generally available at grocery stores. Be sure to purchase the long-cooking type and avoid anything that is labeled quick-cooking.

- Quinoa is available at some grocery stores, heath food stores, and online.

- Yams and sweet potatoes are available at the grocery stores. If you can't find them, ask the produce manager to order some for you.

- You already know where to find cauliflower.

Basmati Rice Pilaf

Yield:	Serving size:	Prep time:	Cook time:
8 servings	$3/8$ cup	15 minutes	20 minutes
Each serving has:			
17 g carbohydrate	1 g fiber	2 g protein	

2 cups water

1 cube chicken bouillon

1 cup brown basmati rice

2 TB. butter

1. Put water and bouillon cube in a microwave-safe bowl or a glass measuring cup and microwave for 4 minutes or until boiling. At the same time, sauté rice in butter in a large saucepan until hot and some kernels start to toast.

2. Put on a potholder mitten that protects your wrist. Turn down the heat to simmer. All at once, pour boiling water over rice and cover. Cook about 20 minutes or until fluffy.

HOT POTATO

Be very careful when you pour the boiling water into the rice, and expect lots of steam and hissing. The pot might even boil over. Be sure to protect your hand. Taking this much care is worth it—the rice is the best ever.

RECIPE FOR SUCCESS

Basmati rice has just as many carbs as regular rice; however, the glycemic index count is lower. So use brown basmati rice because it will keep your blood sugar levels lower than white rice. Use this rice recipe whenever you want a rice accompaniment to your meal.

Pine Nut-Barley Pilaf

Yield:	Serving size:	Prep time:	Cook time:
10 servings	⅓ cup	20 minutes	1 hour, 10 minutes
Each serving has:			
13 g carbohydrate	4 g fiber	3 g protein	

1 cup pearl barley

⅓ cup pine nuts

6 TB. butter

½ cup green onions, chopped

½ cup fresh parsley, chopped

¼ tsp. salt

¼ tsp. freshly ground black pepper

3⅓ cups water or chicken broth

1. Preheat the oven to 350°F.

2. Rinse barley in cold water and drain. In a heavy skillet, sauté pine nuts in butter until toasted. Remove with a slotted spoon and reserve. Sauté green onions with barley until lightly toasted. Remove from heat. Stir in nuts, parsley, salt, and pepper. Put into an ungreased 2-quart oven casserole.

3. Heat water to boiling and pour over barley mixture, blending well. Bake, uncovered, 1 hour, 10 minutes.

RECIPE FOR SUCCESS

This recipe is a nutty tasting accompaniment to main dishes. It makes a filling pilaf, so you feel satisfied with less.

TABLE TALK

Barley is one of two low-glycemic grains. The other is steel-cut oats. Even though pearl barley contains the same amount of carbs as other grains, it doesn't cause a quick rise in blood sugar as other grains do. But eat only limited amounts infrequently.

Baked Yams

Yield:	Serving size:	Prep time:	Cook time:
8 servings	½ yam per person	5 minutes	1 hour

Each serving has:			
16 g carbohydrate	3 g fiber	1 g protein	

4 small yams or 2 large

1. Preheat the oven to 375°F.

2. Wash yams and place directly on cooking rack in the oven. Bake 1 hour or until done.

3. Serve topped with your favorite condiments: salt, pepper, sour cream, butter, chives, bacon, or cinnamon. Based on the condiments you choose, the carbohydrate and protein counts may increase.

RECIPE FOR SUCCESS

Serve with butter and, if you prefer, a sprinkling of cinnamon. They are delicious.

Barley with Dill

Yield:	Serving size:	Prep time:	Cook time:
12 servings	⅓ cup	15 minutes	1½ hours

Each serving has:			
16 g carbohydrate	4 g fiber	5 g protein	

1 small onion, chopped

¼ cup butter

1¾ cups barley

1 tsp. salt

1 tsp. fresh dill

½ tsp. freshly ground black pepper

4 cups water or chicken broth

1. Preheat the oven to 350°F.

2. In a medium saucepan, sauté onion in butter until golden brown. Transfer to a baking dish with a lid. Add barley, salt, dill, pepper, and water. Mix well. Cover and bake 1½ hours.

RECIPE FOR SUCCESS

Barley has lots of texture and plenty of fiber. Use it to accompany pork chops, steak, and other very low-carb main dishes.

Quinoa Pilaf with Vegetables

Yield:	Serving size:	Prep time:	Cook time:
8 servings	½ cup	20 minutes	25 minutes

Each serving has:			
14 g carbohydrate	2 g fiber	6 g protein	

1 cup uncooked quinoa, rinsed

1¾ cups water

2 TB. butter

¼ cup red bell pepper, diced

¼ cup green bell pepper, diced

2 medium carrots, diced

2 celery stalks, diced

1 tsp. garlic, minced

2 TB. grated Parmesan cheese

Salt and freshly ground black pepper to taste

1. In a medium saucepan, combine quinoa and water over medium heat. Bring to a boil, reduce heat, cover, and simmer until quinoa is tender and liquid is absorbed, about 15 minutes. Remove from heat.

2. In a heavy skillet, heat butter and add red and green peppers, carrots, and celery. Cook, stirring, until just soft. Stir in garlic. Cook 1 minute longer.

3. Stir into quinoa. Add Parmesan cheese, salt, and pepper, and mix well. Serve hot.

TABLE TALK

The Incas considered quinoa (pronounced keen-WAUGH) the "mother grain." Find it at the health food store if it isn't available at your grocer. Quinoa is a primitive grain, so enjoy the unique taste in this pilaf. You get 1 serving of vegetables with this pilaf. Serve as a side dish with very low-carb main dishes, such as seafood, meat, or fish.

Cajun Dirty Rice

Yield:	Serving size:	Prep time:	Cook time:
6 servings	¾ cup	30 minutes plus refrigeration time if made in advance	30 minutes

Each serving has:		
21 g carbohydrate	1 g fiber	15 g protein

2 chicken livers	1 red bell pepper, chopped
6 chicken gizzards	3 stalks celery, chopped
3 cups water	2 cloves garlic, minced
1 cup uncooked brown basmati rice	¼ tsp. cayenne
½ lb. ground beef	1 tsp. salt
¼ cup butter	1 bay leaf
½ cup green onions, chopped	½ tsp. thyme
	¼ cup fresh parsley, chopped

1. Boil livers and gizzards in 1 cup water, and set aside to cool. Discard cooking water. Chop livers and gizzards very fine or use a food processor to blend.

2. Cook rice in remaining 2 cups water, adding additional water if needed.

3. In a large heavy skillet, brown ground beef and drain. Remove meat to a side bowl.

4. In the skillet, melt butter and sauté onion, bell pepper, celery, and garlic until vegetables are tender. Add drained meat and mashed livers and gizzards to vegetable mixture and heat. Add cayenne, salt, bay leaf, thyme, and water left from cooking livers and gizzards. Cover and simmer 30 minutes. Remove bay leaf, and add cooked rice. Mix well and add parsley. Serve.

5. This dish freezes well. It is best when it is made 24 hours in advance so the flavors can blend. Reheat in the microwave or a skillet when ready to serve.

RECIPE FOR SUCCESS

You can substitute 1 tablespoon Cajun Spice Mix for spices in the ingredient list. If you do not want to use livers and gizzards, substitute an additional $\frac{1}{2}$ pound ground beef or sausage. Serve with an additional vegetable dish to have a balanced and complete meal.

Green Brown Rice

Yield:	Serving size:	Prep time:	Cook time:
12 servings	$\frac{1}{2}$ cup	20 minutes	40 minutes
Each serving has:			
11 g carbohydrate	1 g fiber	4 g protein	

2 cups cooked brown basmati rice

2 eggs

$\frac{1}{2}$ cup cheddar cheese, grated

$\frac{3}{4}$ cup bell pepper, chopped

$\frac{1}{2}$ cup fresh parsley, chopped

4 green onions, chopped

2 cups Basic Cream Soup (see recipe in Chapter 14)

1 jalapeño pepper, chopped

1 TB. red wine vinegar

1 TB. Cajun Spice Mix (see Chapter 12)

1. Preheat the oven to 350°F. Grease a large casserole baking pan.

2. In a large bowl, combine rice, eggs, cheese, bell pepper, parsley, green onions, soup, jalapeño, vinegar, and Cajun Spice Mix, and pour into the baking pan. Cover and bake 30 to 40 minutes until bubbly. Remove cover and stir well. This dish freezes well.

RECIPE FOR SUCCESS

You can add frozen or steamed broccoli or other green veggies to this dish; add cream or water if adding vegetables. This makes a wonderful vegetable to take to a covered-dish event, as it is just as delicious at room temperature as it is piping hot.

Jalapeño Red Potato Bowls

Yield:	Serving size:	Prep time:	Cook time:
6 servings	2 halves	20 minutes	15 minutes
Each serving has:			
5 g carbohydrate	1 g fiber	2 g protein	

6 small new red potatoes, halved

¼ tsp. cayenne

Salt to taste

1 TB. olive oil

1 (3-oz.) pkg. cream cheese, softened

1 jalapeño pepper, finely chopped

1 TB. pimiento, chopped

2 slices bacon, cooked until crisp, chopped

1. Preheat the oven to 400°F.

2. Toss potato halves with cayenne, salt, and oil. Place cut side down on a greased baking pan. Bake about 15 minutes until cooked through.

3. Scoop out flesh, leaving a bit around edge.

4. Meanwhile, place cream cheese, jalapeño, pimiento, and potato flesh into a small food processor or an electric mixer. Blend well. Fill each potato bowl with cream cheese mixture, and garnish with chopped bacon.

Mock Mashed Potatoes

Yield:	Serving size:	Prep time:	Cook time:
6 servings	½ cup	10 minutes	5 minutes

Each serving has:		
2 g carbohydrate	1 g fiber	1 g protein

3 cups cauliflower, chopped

1 TB. butter

¼ cup sour cream

Salt and freshly ground black pepper to taste

1. Microwave cauliflower and butter until soft enough to mash. Place cauliflower in a food processor with sour cream, and process until the texture of mashed potatoes. Stir in salt and pepper and serve.

RECIPE FOR SUCCESS

A delicious lower-carb substitute for real mashed potatoes, cauliflower makes terrific mashed "potatoes." Feel free to add garlic powder and cheese to give more flavor if not serving with gravy.

Mock Potato Salad

Yield:	Serving size:	Prep time:	Cook time:
6 servings	½ cup	15 minutes plus chill time	None

Each serving has:		
3 g carbohydrate	1 g fiber	4 g protein

3 cups cauliflower florets, cut into bite-size pieces

6 TB. green onion, chopped

1 cup celery, chopped

6 TB. bell pepper, chopped

3 hard-boiled eggs, chopped

1 tsp. garlic, minced

1 tsp. dill weed

½ tsp. dry mustard

¾ cup mayonnaise

2 TB. sour cream

Paprika, for garnish

1. Combine cauliflower, green onion, celery, bell pepper, eggs, garlic, dill weed, mustard, mayonnaise, and sour cream and chill. Add a sprinkle of paprika just before serving.

RECIPE FOR SUCCESS

No one will ever know this recipe doesn't contain potatoes! Cauliflower makes a great potato substitute. You can lightly steam the cauliflower for about 3 minutes if you prefer your salad with less crunch. For extra protein, add 8 ounces firm tofu cut into ½-inch cubes or small cubes of any favorite cheese.

Twice-Baked Potatoes

Yield:	Serving size:	Prep time:	Cook time:
6 servings	½ potato	15 minutes	1 hour, 20 minutes
Each serving has:			
16 g carbohydrate	4 g fiber	2 g protein	

3 medium sweet potatoes

¼ cup cream

¼ tsp. ground nutmeg

¼ tsp. ground cinnamon

¼ tsp. ground cloves

2 TB. pecans, chopped

6 tsp. butter

1. Preheat the oven to 375°F.

2. Scrub potatoes. Place on a baking pan, and bake 1 hour or until done. Remove from the oven. Let stand until cool enough to handle.

3. Slice potatoes in half, and remove flesh from skins, keeping skins intact. Place flesh into a bowl, and keep skins on the baking pan. Set aside skins until ready to fill.

4. Mix cream, nutmeg, cinnamon, and cloves with potato flesh and mash well. Scoop potato mixture back into shells, and bake 20 minutes until hot.

5. Sprinkle with pecans, and serve with butter pat melting on top.

RECIPE FOR SUCCESS

This dish is a much lower-carb relative of traditional white potatoes. The mashed sweet potato can also be served without restuffing the skins, if desired.

Sweet Potato Oven Fries

Yield:	Serving size:	Prep time:	Cook time:
6 servings	½ potato	15 minutes	30 minutes

Each serving has:			
16 g carbohydrate	3 g fiber	1 g protein	

3 sweet potatoes
1 tsp. melted butter

½ tsp. salt
Additional favorite seasonings
   as desired

1. Preheat the oven to 450°F.

2. Line a baking dish with foil. Wash potatoes and cut into wedges.

3. In a large bowl, toss potato wedges with melted butter, salt, and seasonings.
   Spread potatoes on the foil in a single layer, and bake 20 minutes. Loosen
   potatoes from the pan, and turn to roast 10 minutes longer or until done.

RECIPE FOR SUCCESS

Although potatoes are a higher-carb food, the sweet potatoes cause less of a
rise in blood sugar than white potatoes. These make a nice treat every once in a
while, and you know they are a lot healthier than fried potatoes!

The Least You Need to Know

- Potatoes and grains can fit into a low-carb eating plan.
- Sweet potatoes, yams, and cauliflower are excellent alternatives to white
  potatoes—and are more delicious.
- Using whole low-glycemic grains is a healthy and delicious way to eat low carb.
- These foods are naturally higher in carbs, so follow serving size suggestions
  carefully.

Desserts

In This Chapter

- The sweet ending of a meal
- Sweet, yummy, *and* low carb
- Your comfort foods
- Tastes like high carb

You have taste buds that signal "sweet," which means your body seeks out sweet foods to satisfy the taste buds. It's not totally accurate to say you have a sweet tooth as it is to say your sweet taste buds want satisfaction. As humans, it's natural to want to eat something sweet. In fact, your taste buds cause you to seek out all five taste sensations, so it's important to balance sweet with the other four—sour, salt, bitter, and umami (protein).

Though we usually eat desserts at the end of a meal, you can eat dessert first. But make sure when you do that you save room in your stomach for the main course. As children, we learned to save room for desserts. Some of us were required to clean our plates before our parents permitted us to eat dessert. Because of this, dessert may not be as fattening as the "cleaning your plate" requirement.

Hurrah! Now desserts can be low carb without sacrificing flavor, the comfort factor, and satisfying ingredients. In fact, these desserts are so yummy that you can serve them with pride to your family and guests, and they won't even know they're eating low carb, which is just as it should be.

Desserts as Comfort Foods

Comfort foods, put quite simply, are any foods that make us feel good. Somehow, almost inexplicably, they elicit feelings of being loved and accepted, like a tail-wagging puppy who greets us when we get home. We turn to comfort foods when stressed, anxious, and under pressure, and they deliver short-term results.

Desserts are listed among all-time favorite comfort foods. The good news is that you don't have to give them up, because in this chapter, you'll find cookies, puddings, mousses, cheesecake, and even ice cream!

So you can have it all—comfort foods plus healthy, low-carb eating.

Ingredients

Use high-quality ingredients for your desserts. High-quality ingredients contribute to taste and texture and to your ultimate satisfaction.

- **Nuts.** Use the freshest you can purchase. Many grocery and health food stores now offer bulk nuts, and the prices are lower than the small packages of nuts offered in the baking section. Keep nuts fresh by storing them in the refrigerator.

- **Heavy cream or whipping cream.** If you need to use a less-rich substitute, try frozen whipped topping.

- **Cheese.** Use regular cheese, not low-fat cheese. Using low-fat products increases the carb count of the recipe and sacrifices quality and taste.

- **Sugar.** The recipes call for small amounts sugar. Of all the available sweeteners, it is the least controversial. Most people can tolerate sugar in small amounts. If you don't want to use sugar, you can substitute sucralose (brand name Splenda) or Truvia. Both types of sugar substitute have fewer carbs. Don't substitute aspartame for sugar in a recipe that is baked or heated, because it doesn't hold up well to heat. Nothing satisfies a person's sweet tooth like the natural real sweeteners—honey, sugar, and fruit.

- **Molasses.** Choose dark molasses for a stronger taste and light molasses if you prefer a milder taste. Molasses adds a caramel brown sugar flavor to the dessert. A little molasses goes a long way, thus the recipe has fewer carbs than brown sugar.

HOT POTATO

If you are having intense and constant sugar cravings, chances are good that you don't need more sugar. Most likely, you need more complete protein for both breakfast and lunch. Protein keeps blood sugar levels stable throughout the day and prevents the drop in blood sugar that leads to insatiable sugar cravings. The rule of thumb for your daily protein intake is to divide your weight in pounds by 2. So if you weigh 150 pounds, you need 75 grams of protein. It's best if you get ⅓ of that amount at each meal. For example, ⅓ of 75 is 25. So get 25 grams protein at each meal.

Low-Carbing Any Dessert Recipe

If you have a favorite dessert recipe and want to make it low carb, try some of these suggestions. Remember that the type of recipe will make a big difference in your success. In most dessert recipes, the sugar and flour contribute the most carbs.

- Sugar is high in carbs, with 200 in 1 cup. In most recipes, you can halve the amount of sugar and not even notice it.

- White, all-purpose flour has 95 carbs per cup; whole wheat has 87. When you can, eliminate the flour altogether by substituting almond or pecan "flour." Flour or cornstarch is the unequalled best for thickening sauces, so don't substitute a nut flour here. But usually, if the recipe calls for 2 tablespoons flour or cornstarch, you can get great results with only 1 tablespoon. Substituting nut flour for wheat flour in cakes made with baking powder or baking soda may or may not work well. You be the judge.

- Upgrade milk to heavy cream. One cup milk has 50 carbs; 1 cup cream has 7.

Creating a new recipe out of an old one requires working through trial and error, learning from your mistakes, and trying again until you get it right. That's why they call them "test kitchens." And sometimes even the errors taste good enough to eat.

Even Lower Carbs

Because these are dessert recipes, they have a higher carbohydrate count than other types of food, such as fruits, vegetables, and meat.

If you really want something sweet but the carb counts of the desserts would cause you to exceed your daily quota, eat half a serving. You'll eat half the carbs and still satisfy your sweet tooth.

Raspberry Mousse

Yield:	Serving size:	Prep time:	Cook time:
10 servings	1 custard cup	30 minutes plus chill time	None

Each serving has:		
8 g carbohydrate	4 g fiber	2 g protein

1 TB. or 1 envelope unflavored gelatin	2 large egg yolks
2 TB. cold water	3 TB. sugar
¼ cup orange juice	2 cups heavy cream
2 (10-oz.) bags frozen raspberries, unsweetened	Sprigs fresh mint, or fresh fruit for garnish

1. Soak gelatin in cold water in a saucepan for 5 minutes. Add orange juice and raspberries, and bring just to boiling, stirring constantly. Cool to room temperature.

2. Beat egg yolks and sugar in a bowl until pale yellow. Put egg yolk mixture into the top pan of a double boiler over simmering water. Stir until slightly thickened. Cool to room temperature.

3. Add egg yolk mixture to raspberry mixture. Stir until blended. Whip heavy cream into soft peaks, and fold into egg yolk and raspberry mixture. Divide among 10 small custard-type dishes and chill.

4. Garnish with fresh mint sprigs or fresh fruit. Serve chilled.

Variation: You can substitute any kind of fresh or unsweetened frozen berries—strawberries, blackberries, or blueberries. The carbohydrate count stays about the same.

RECIPE FOR SUCCESS

This recipe has great mouth appeal. The tart taste of the berries, the rich cream, and some sugar simply feels good all over.

Tapioca Pudding

Yield:	Serving size:	Prep time:	Cook time:
8 servings	About ⅓ cup	5 minutes plus chill time	15 minutes

Each serving has:		
14 g carbohydrate	0 g fiber	3 g protein

3 TB. quick-cooking tapioca

¼ cup sugar

¼ tsp. salt

2 large eggs, beaten

2 cups whole milk

½ tsp. vanilla extract

1. Combine tapioca, sugar, salt, eggs, and milk. Without stirring, cook in the top of a double boiler over boiling water for 7 minutes. Continue to cook, stirring, for 5 more minutes. Remove from heat, stir in vanilla, and let cool. Chill.

RECIPE FOR SUCCESS

Pudding is an old-fashioned comfort food and is low in carbs. You can even sprinkle toasted almonds or coconut over the pudding and still have a relatively low-carb dessert. But be careful about serving size with the dessert recipes. A second serving can overload you with too many carbs.

Crustless Cheesecake

Yield:	Serving size:	Prep time:	Cook time:
12 servings	1 slice	15 minutes	50 minutes
Each serving has:			
7 g carbohydrate	0 g fiber	7 g protein	

1 cup 4 percent fat cottage cheese	4 large eggs
1 (8-oz.) pkg. regular cream cheese, softened (not light)	2 TB. lemon juice
	6 TB. brown sugar
1 cup sour cream	

1. Preheat the oven to 350°F.

2. Combine cottage cheese, cream cheese, sour cream, eggs, lemon juice, and brown sugar in a blender, and pulse until well blended. Pour into a lightly greased 8-inch springform pan, and bake for 50 minutes. Cool. Slice into 12 servings.

Variation: Because this cheesecake is plain and unadorned, you can add fruit or a favorite topping. But remember that a topping can increase the carbohydrate count.

HOT POTATO

Be sure to use full-fat cottage cheese, sour cream, and cream cheese. If you use low-fat products, the carb count could double and the taste won't be as delicious.

Slow Cooker Country Apples

Yield:	Serving size:	Prep time:	Cook time:
6 servings	¾ cup	10 minutes	4 to 6 hours
Each serving has:			
19 g carbohydrate	3 g fiber	1 g protein	

4 cups Granny Smith or Golden Delicious apples, peeled and sliced

⅓ cup raisins

¼ tsp. cinnamon

¼ cup slow-cooking oatmeal, raw

1 cup water

½ cup apple juice

3 TB. butter

1. In a slow cooker, stir together apples, raisins, cinnamon, and oatmeal. Add water and apple juice. Stir. Dot with pieces of butter. Cook on low 4 to 6 hours.

Rum-Flavored Bananas

Yield:	Serving size:	Prep time:	Cook time:
6 servings	½ banana	10 minutes	10 minutes
Each serving has:			
9 g carbohydrate	1 g fiber	< 1 g protein	

2 bananas, peeled and sliced lengthwise

2 TB. butter

¼ cup rum

Whipped cream (optional)

1. Cut each lengthwise piece banana crosswise to make 4 pieces from each banana. Melt butter in a skillet, and toss bananas until warm; add rum and heat until hot. Remove from heat, and carefully ignite rum with a long match. Rotate pan from side to side while flaming. This allows alcohol to cook out.

2. Serve while hot. Add a dollop whipped cream (if using).

HOT POTATO

Be cautious when flaming alcohol. Be sure the rum is hot before trying to light or it may not flame. A good safety tip would be to wear protective eye glasses or turn your head when lighting the alcohol. Definitely use a long match.

RECIPE FOR SUCCESS

Of course this sauce is delicious over ice cream! Just remember to check the ice-cream label and count additional carbohydrates. Use other fruits instead of bananas such as peaches, cooked apples, pitted cherries, or mixed fruits. If soft fruits are too ripe, they tend to melt away during the flaming.

Strawberry Cream

Yield:	Serving size:	Prep time:	Cook time:
6 servings	½ cup	15 minutes	None

Each serving has:			
6 g carbohydrate	< 1 g fiber	< 1 g protein	

1½ cups heavy cream

¼ cup low-carb strawberry fruit preserves, at room temperature

½ tsp. almond or vanilla extract (optional)

Mint leaves, for garnish (optional)

1. Pour heavy cream into ice-cold bowl, and whip until thick and creamy. Lightly stir in preserves. If additional flavor is desired, add almond extract.

2. Serve in small dessert dishes topped with mint leaf (if using) or use 2 tablespoons as a luscious topping on fresh fruit or Double Chocolate Brownies (see recipe in Chapter 25).

RECIPE FOR SUCCESS

Substitute any flavor of fruit preserves for the strawberry. But read the label on the jar for no more than 6 grams carbohydrate per serving; avoid those made with sugar substitutes.

Hot Fruit Soufflé

Yield:	Serving size:	Prep time:	Cook time:
6 servings	½ cup	30 minutes	25 minutes
Each serving has:			
6 g carbohydrate	1 g fiber	4 g protein	

2 cups fresh fruit, your choice

1 TB. honey

2 large egg yolks, at room temperature

2 TB. heavy cream

5 large egg whites, at room temperature

Pinch salt

1. Preheat the oven to 350°F.

2. In a food processor, combine fruit, honey, egg yolks, and cream. Process well.

3. In a separate bowl, beat egg whites with pinch of salt until very stiff peaks form. Fold in fruit mixture quickly but gently. Pour fruit mixture into a buttered 1-quart soufflé dish, and bake about 25 minutes.

4. Do *not* open the oven door during baking or soufflé could fall. Serve immediately.

HOT POTATO

This recipe can be doubled and made in a larger soufflé dish. It can be made in several smaller soufflé cups if individual servings are desired.

RECIPE FOR SUCCESS

What a delightful ending to a meal—this light refreshing dessert is delicious following any of the heavier main courses. Fresh berries make a wonderful soufflé. If desired, use unsweetened frozen berries, but bring them to room temperature first. If frozen with sugar, you won't need the honey, but you may need to adjust the carbohydrate count. You can use dried fruit, but cook it first in a small amount of water to soften. Let cool before using.

Peanut Butter Cookies

Yield:	Serving size:	Prep time:	Cook time:
20 servings	1 cookie	10 minutes	10 minutes
Each serving has:			
7 g carbohydrate	1 g fiber	4 g protein	

½ cup natural peanut butter, no sugar added

½ cup sugar

1 tsp. molasses

¼ cup heavy cream

½ cup almonds, slivered

½ tsp. baking powder

1½ cups almond flour (1¼ cups almonds, finely ground)

½ tsp. salt

2 tsp. vanilla extract

1. Preheat the oven to 375°F.

2. Mix together peanut butter, sugar, molasses, cream, almonds, baking powder, almond flour, salt, and vanilla, and drop by teaspoonfuls onto a greased cookie sheet to make 20 cookies. If you prefer, press cookies with the tines of a fork for that peanut-butter-cookie checkerboard look. Bake about 10 to 12 minutes or until set.

RECIPE FOR SUCCESS

We couldn't tell these were low carb. They will surely satisfy your sweet tooth. Add to sack lunches or as an after-school or after-work snack.

TABLE TALK

You can easily make almond flour with a food processor and almonds. Use either blanched or unblanched whole almonds. To make 1 cup almond flour, use about ¾ cup whole almonds and process until the almonds turn into a fluffy powder. Be sure to watch carefully—don't process so long that you make almond butter. You can also purchase almond flour online.

Gingersnaps

Yield:	Serving size:	Prep time:	Cook time:
24 servings	1 cookie	10 minutes	20 minutes

Each serving has:		
5 g carbohydrate	1 g fiber	2 g protein

½ cup butter (1 stick)

½ cup sugar

1 TB. molasses

1 large egg

2 tsp. freshly grated ginger or 1 tsp. ground ginger

1 tsp. cinnamon

¼ tsp. nutmeg

¼ tsp. cloves

½ tsp. salt

2 cups almond flour (1½ cups almonds, finely ground)

1. Preheat the oven to 300°F.

2. Cream butter with sugar and molasses. Beat in egg. Add ginger, cinnamon, nutmeg, cloves, and salt and mix. Gradually add almond flour, and mix to a stiff dough. Form into 24 small balls, and place on a greased cookie sheet about 1 inch apart. Bake for 20 minutes.

Variation: If you like the taste of ginger without the other spices, increase the amount of ginger to 3 teaspoons and omit the nutmeg, cinnamon, and cloves.

RECIPE FOR SUCCESS

Enjoy the aroma of fresh gingerbread when baking these cookies. And they taste just as good. Why not roll or mold dough into gingerbread men?

Baked Ricotta Cups

Yield:	Serving size:	Prep time:	Cook time:
8 servings	1 cup	15 minutes	20 minutes

Each serving has:		
8 g carbohydrate	1 g fiber	5 g protein

1 cup ricotta cheese

2 large egg whites, beaten

1 TB. honey

3 cups mixed fresh or frozen fruit (such as strawberries, peaches, raspberries, blackberries, or cherries; pitted)

1. Preheat the oven to 350°F.

2. Place ricotta cheese into a bowl, and break it up with a wooden spoon. Add beaten egg whites and honey, and mix thoroughly until smooth and well blended.

3. Lightly grease 8 ramekins. Spoon ricotta mixture into the prepared ramekins, and bake for 20 minutes until ricotta cakes rise and are golden.

4. Meanwhile, place fruit in a pan with a little water if fruit is fresh, and heat gently until softened. Let cool slightly, and remove any pits if using cherries. Serve fruit sauce over ricotta cups.

RECIPE FOR SUCCESS

The ricotta cups look elegant, yet are quite easy to make and are a great dessert for any time of year. Expect the berries to be slightly tart—it just adds to the intense fresh-fruit taste. Serve the fruit sauce warm or chilled.

Cherry Omelet

Yield:	Serving size:	Prep time:	Cook time:
8 servings	⅙ omelet	10 minutes plus 10 minutes to pit cherries	6 minutes

Each serving has:			
10 g carbohydrate	1 g fiber	6 g protein	

1 pint or 2 cups fresh or frozen cherries, pitted	¼ cup sugar
8 TB. butter	4 tsp. rum
8 large eggs	Pinch salt

1. Remove stems and stones from cherries, and sauté for 5 minutes in 4 table-spoons butter. Beat eggs hard with sugar, rum, and salt. Add cherries to batter.

2. Heat remaining 4 tablespoons butter in a skillet or fold-over omelet pan. Tilt the pan so butter coats sides of the pan all the way to the top to prevent omelet from sticking. Set the pan over medium-low heat. Pour batter into the skillet or half batter into each side of the omelet pan. With a spatula, push batter in from the sides to allow top, uncooked egg to run over to the pan. When eggs are set on bottom, fold over omelet or close the fold-over pan.

RECIPE FOR SUCCESS

The cherries in this omelet will make you forget everything you've ever heard about omelets being only for breakfast. It tastes totally indulgent.

Frozen Raspberry Soufflé

Yield:	Serving size:	Prep time:	Cook time:
10 servings	⅓ cup	20 minutes plus chill time	1 hour

Each serving has:			
21 g carbohydrate	1 g fiber	3 g protein	

¾ cup sugar

¼ cup water

8 large egg yolks

2 cups heavy whipping cream

1 cup fresh or unsweetened frozen raspberries

1. Boil ¾ cup sugar and water to make a hot syrup. Boil until the hot syrup falls in a long thread from the spoon or registers 220°F on a candy thermometer, about 5 to 8 minutes.

2. Beat egg yolks lightly with a fork in the top of a double boiler. Slowly add hot syrup, stirring constantly with a wooden spoon. Cook in the top of a double boiler for 45 minutes, stirring frequently until sauce has consistency of thin mayonnaise.

3. Whip cream. Crush raspberries with a fork, and mix with whipped cream.

4. Combine mixtures and mix well. Pour into individual ramekins, or long-stemmed wine or champagne glasses. You can also pour into a bowl and serve family-style. Chill thoroughly.

RECIPE FOR SUCCESS

This recipe is truly elegant for a dinner party, but you'll enjoy leftovers the next day.

Sautéed Fruit

Yield:	Serving size:	Prep time:	Cook time:
8 servings	¾ cup	15 minutes	15 minutes

Each serving has:		
14 g carbohydrate	3 g fiber	1 g protein

2 apples, peeled, cored, and cut into thick slices (your choice)

1 pear, peeled, cored, and cut into thick slices

1½ TB. fresh lemon juice

3 TB. butter

2 TB. orange marmalade

1 TB. Grand Marnier

2 navel oranges, peeled and sectioned

Sprigs of fresh mint (optional)

1. In a small bowl, toss apple and pear slices with lemon juice. In a large skillet, melt 2 tablespoons butter, add fruit, and sauté over medium-high heat until apples are tender, stirring gently.

2. With a slotted spoon, transfer fruit mixture to a bowl. To the skillet, add marmalade, Grand Marnier, and remaining 1 tablespoon butter. Stir until melted. Pour sauce over fruit, add oranges and toss gently. Garnish with sprigs of mint.

RECIPE FOR SUCCESS

This recipe is a delicious way to dress up these fruits, and they are available fresh year-round! The sauce would be dreamy served over sponge cake with or without the fruit if you have enough carbs left in your daily allotment.

Cold Lemon and Blueberry Mousse

Yield:	Serving size:	Prep time:	Cook time:
6 servings	About ⅔ cup	25 minutes plus chill time	None

Each serving has:		
23 g carbohydrate	1 g fiber	5 g protein

5 large egg yolks

½ cup sugar

¼ cup fresh lemon juice

5 large egg whites, beaten stiff

2 cups (1 pint) fresh or frozen blueberries

1. Beat egg yolks with sugar until light and lemon-colored. Add lemon juice and mix well. Stir over hot water in the top of a double boiler until thick. Remove from heat, and fold in egg whites. Carefully fold in blueberries. Pour into a serving dish, and chill in refrigerator for at least 1 hour.

Variation: Substitute blackberries or raspberries in this recipe, or omit the berries entirely and enjoy the singular refreshing taste of lemon.

RECIPE FOR SUCCESS

The blueberries add color and eye appeal and are a great way to balance the lemon flavor. Plus, all berries provide wonderful nutrition and antioxidants. Serve with mint garnish.

The Least You Need to Know

- The sweet taste buds on your tongue like to be satisfied with desserts and sweet-tasting foods.
- Low-carb desserts are a tasty, sweet ending to a meal.
- Eat your comfort foods in comfort, knowing they are low carb.
- Low-carb desserts don't have to taste low carb.
- You can modify your favorite desserts to be low carb with some experimentation.

Chocolate

In This Chapter

- A luscious, sometimes decadent, low-carb treat
- Choosing types of chocolate
- Nutritional value
- Getting picky about your chocolate

Chocolate is a gift from the gods, or so the pre-Columbian Central American natives believed. Because of its richness, exotic flavor, and intensity, chocolate was used in the ceremonies honoring the Mayan and Aztec gods. It was a drink worthy of the king and nobility. They seasoned their chocolate drinks with peppers, vanilla, anise seeds, and corn. Ancient records indicate they used chocolate for religious rituals, for currency, for increasing stamina, and for daily refreshment.

Today, many of us still hold chocolate in similar high esteem. We think chocolate feeds our souls, our energy, and our hearts. It represents dreams of romance, reconciliation, and eternal love.

The reality of chocolate isn't so bad, either. It can easily fit into an overall low-carb diet. Chocolate is packed with antioxidants and other good-for-you nutrition. To honor its culinary and sensuous pleasures, chocolate has its own chapter of recipes in this book. Whether you are an avowed chocoholic, simply fond of the taste, or need a daily "fix," you can find what you are looking for—low-carb chocolate delights—right here.

Eat Your Chocolate—It's Good for You

Chocolate is actually beneficial for you. Recent studies show that its powerful antioxidants can help prevent cancer and heart disease. It even fights tooth decay! And just think, for years we thought it gave us cavities.

The cocoa bean contains antioxidants, stearic acid, magnesium, calcium, and caffeine. These plus about 300 other substances create the flavor and nutritional value of chocolate.

Chocolate contains catechins and phenols, antioxidants that are indicated in the prevention of cancer and heart disease. Until recently, experts thought tea had the highest concentration of these great disease fighters, but now we know dark chocolate has four times more.

The phenols in chocolate are like those in red wine. They protect against heart disease and reduce day-to-day damage to cells and DNA from free radicals. They also prevent fatlike substances in the bloodstream from oxidizing and clogging the arteries. Along with all this, chocolate helps thwart mouth bacteria and stop dental decay. We must have intuitively sensed this all along as we ate our chocolate!

TABLE TALK

We can't imagine a worthy substitute for chocolate. In our guilt-ridden days of thinking it made us fat, we tried carob. It wasn't the same. So don't even think of using another ingredient in place of chocolate. If you did, the recipe wouldn't come close to being a food fit for the god or goddess in you.

But, a little goes a long way. You don't need to eat a lot of chocolate to enjoy the benefits. You also can obtain similar benefits from fruits and vegetables. But it's nice to know you get value from eating chocolate. As dark chocolate is the most beneficial type for your health, most recipes in this chapter call for dark or bitter chocolate.

Chocolate Choices

The varieties of chocolate are seemingly endless. You can purchase the least expensive at the store and create a wonderful dessert, or you can use the most expensive you can find, perhaps on the Internet, and enjoy extraordinary taste and aroma.

Here are some recommendations:

- **Cocoa powder (unsweetened).** For these recipes we've used both Hershey's baking cocoa in the famous dark brown tin and Ghiradelli cocoa powder we purchased at the health food store. Hershey's has a stronger taste. Ghiradelli is milder and softer. Be sure that when the recipe calls for cocoa powder you don't use the sweetened kind.

- **Alkaline processed cocoa powder.** You can substitute this powder for cocoa powder in these recipes. It makes the dessert darker in color. The flavor will be less tangy or acidic, so expect a smoother, softer taste.

- **Unsweetened baking chocolate squares.** You can substitute cocoa powder for the squares by using 3 tablespoons cocoa powder plus 1 tablespoon butter for each square.

- **Chocolate morsels.** Today, you can obtain excellent quality chocolate as chocolate chips. We like our chocolate deep, creamy, and flavorful. Our preferences are Ghiradelli semisweet and double chocolate morsels and Guittard milk chocolate, and semisweet morsels.

- **Chocolate bars.** You can substitute a good-quality chocolate bar such as Choco-love, Ghiradelli, or Guittard in many of the recipes. We have found the best quality and most variety at some grocery stores, health food stores, and at cooking supply stores. You can now purchase high-quality chocolate in 10-pound bars, which is quite economical. To break up the bars into chocolate chunks or morsels, we suggest this: Unwrap the chocolate bar and place it in a plastic zippered bag. Take it to the front or back porch and drop it on the concrete. Any remaining chunks that are too large you can break up by hand.

Most grocery stores offer a good selection of chips and cocoa powders in the baking, spice, and flour aisle. For fancier brands of chocolate, try the larger health food grocery stores and specialty grocers and cooking stores.

TABLE TALK

Chocolate can burn very easily. To melt, use one of these two methods: place the broken-up chocolate in a dish and microwave on medium for 30 seconds at a time until the chocolate is melted. If you prefer to melt on top of the stove, melt in the top of a double boiler over boiling water.

The Other Ingredients

Chocolate by itself, as found in cocoa powder or bitter baking chocolate, has very few carbs. For most of us, those forms of chocolate are not palatable; in fact, they're unbearable. We need to add sugar and/or dairy products. But even with sugar added, chocolate's carb count is low enough to be considered low carb when you eat moderate amounts.

The recipes in this book call for full-fat dairy products. To get the best results, use real butter, real cream, real cream cheese, and real ricotta cheese. Low-fat dairy products could give you good results, but they may not. Besides, when you use low-fat dairy products, you increase the carbohydrate count of the recipe.

Don't use margarine or fake butter. You'll ruin a good recipe and good chocolate; And the texture and taste won't be as delectable.

Chocolate Carbohydrates

The Aztecs drank hot chocolate made by mixing ground chocolate beans with hot chili peppers, water, and other spices. It was only after the Aztecs served Hernán Cortés this chocolate drink that it was brought to Europe. It's thought that the Spanish first added sugar to their "hot cocoa." They were the first to add carbs to chocolate.

Today, we add not only sugar, but also flour, milk, and other carb-containing ingredients to make delicious desserts. If you want to eat even fewer carbs than the recipe serving size offers, eat a half serving, thus halving the number of carbs you consume. Or you can purchase a dark chocolate candy bar and eat only one square to get that fabulous chocolate taste with very few carbs. And the good news—a bar could last a week or more—as $\frac{1}{4}$ ounce dark chocolate has only 4 carbs.

Double Chocolate Brownies

Yield:	Serving size:	Prep time:	Cook time:
12 servings	1 brownie	10 minutes	20 to 25 minutes

Each serving has:			
10 g carbohydrate	2 g fiber	3 g protein	

$\frac{1}{2}$ cup butter (1 stick)

$\frac{1}{2}$ cup brown sugar

2 large eggs

$\frac{1}{4}$ cup unsweetened cocoa powder

$\frac{3}{4}$ cup ground pecans

$\frac{1}{4}$ tsp. salt

$\frac{1}{2}$ cup dark chocolate chips, either semisweet or double chocolate

1. Preheat the oven to 350°F.

2. Cream butter and brown sugar in a mixing bowl. Beat eggs in well. Add cocoa powder, pecans, and salt. Stir in chocolate chips.

3. Bake in an ungreased 9 × 9-inch pan for 20 to 25 minutes or until done. Cool. Cut into 12 brownies.

Variation: Vary the recipe by adding ¹⁄₂ teaspoon black pepper, 1 teaspoon instant coffee, ¹⁄₄ teaspoon cayenne, or ¹⁄₂ teaspoon vanilla extract. You can also add whole nuts or vary the type of chocolate chips by substituting milk chocolate, white chocolate, or butterscotch chips. You can even try mint chips. However, using these other kinds of chips will increase the carb count.

TABLE TALK

To make ground pecans, use a food processor or a blender. With a food processor, use ¾ cup pecan halves and process until you get a flour. The yield is 1 cup ground pecans. If you use a blender, do not process too long or you will end up with pecan butter. If by chance, you do get pecan butter, it is great on raw vegetables and also eaten with a spoon as a low-carb snack.

Chocolate Soufflé

Yield:	Serving size:	Prep time:	Cook time:
6 servings	¹⁄₆ recipe	20 minutes	12 to 17 minutes
Each serving has:			
11 g carbohydrate	1 g fiber	6 g protein	

4 oz. semisweet or bittersweet chocolate	1 tsp. orange zest, grated
5 TB. butter	1 tsp. sugar
4 large eggs, separated	¹⁄₄ tsp. cream of tartar

1. Preheat the oven to 475°F.

2. Heat chocolate and butter in a saucepan over low heat until chocolate melts. Remove from heat, and stir in egg yolks. Pour into a large mixing bowl, and add grated orange peel.

3. Beat egg whites with 1 teaspoon sugar and cream of tartar until stiff. Fold half beaten egg whites into chocolate mixture. Add remaining whites, and fold in with a spatula. Pour into a greased soufflé dish.

4. Bake 5 minutes; turn temperature down to 425°F, and continue baking for 5 to 7 minutes. Serve immediately.

RECIPE FOR SUCCESS

Soufflés only seem hard to make until you try your first one. Even if it doesn't puff up perfectly, the results are definitely worth eating. This soufflé has a creamy center. If you want it to be less creamy, increase baking time by 4 to 5 minutes.

Chocolate Nut Pâté

Yield:	Serving size:	Prep time:	Cook time:
20 servings	1 small slice	15 minutes plus overnight freezing	5 minutes

Each serving has:		
15 g carbohydrate	1 g fiber	1 g protein

1 (15-oz.) bag semisweet, bitter-sweet, or milk chocolate	4 large egg yolks
1 cup heavy cream	½ cup confectioners' sugar
4 TB. butter	4 TB. dark rum
	½ cup slivered almonds

1. In a heavy saucepan, slowly melt chocolate with cream and butter. Remove from heat, and beat with a wire whisk until smooth. Add egg yolks, one at a time, beating well after each. Add confectioners' sugar, stirring constantly until smooth. Mix in rum. Stir in almonds.

2. Pour mixture into a small 4-cup loaf pan lined with waxed paper. Freeze overnight. To remove pâté, invert pan over a serving plate, and remove waxed paper. Slice and serve.

Variation: In place of the almonds, you can use cashews, pecans, walnuts, macadamias, pistachios, or pine nuts.

RECIPE FOR SUCCESS

This highly rich dessert has the texture of fudge and can be garnished with fresh fruit, such as berries, kiwi, or peaches. You can also serve it topped with whipped cream.

Flourless Chocolate Tiramisu Cake

Yield:	Serving size:	Prep time:	Cook time:
12 servings	$\frac{1}{12}$ cake	20 minutes	30 minutes

Each serving has:			
9 g carbohydrate	2 g fiber	3 g protein	

2 tsp. butter	$\frac{1}{2}$ cup sugar
$\frac{1}{2}$ cup unsweetened cocoa powder	$\frac{1}{2}$ cup sour cream
4 large eggs	1 tsp. vanilla
$\frac{1}{2}$ cup ground hazelnuts	2 tsp. instant coffee

1. Preheat the oven to 350°F.

2. Prepare an 8- or 9-inch springform pan with butter and 1 tablespoon cocoa powder.

3. Using an electric mixer, beat eggs until fluffy and light. In another bowl, combine remaining cocoa powder, hazelnuts, sugar, sour cream, vanilla, and coffee. Carefully fold into beaten egg mixture. Pour into prepared pan.

4. Bake for 30 minutes or until cake is dry on top. Cool until warm. Loosen the edges of cake with a knife, and remove sides of the pan.

Variation: For a plain chocolate cake, omit the coffee. To enhance the flavor of the chocolate, add $\frac{1}{2}$ teaspoon tarragon to the batter.

RECIPE FOR SUCCESS

Be sure to gently and carefully fold the chocolate mixture into the eggs. The cake may sink, but this is normal. Garnish with fresh fruit or whipped cream.

Chocolate Mousse

Yield:	Serving size:	Prep time:	Cook time:
8 servings	⅓ cup	20 minutes plus chill time	None

Each serving has:		
16 g carbohydrate	1 g fiber	4 g protein

2 cups whole milk	4 egg yolks
¼ cup sugar	½ cup whipping cream
½ cup semisweet chocolate morsels	1 tsp. vanilla extract

1. Heat milk, sugar, and chocolate in a saucepan over low heat, stirring until chocolate is melted. Set aside and partially cool. Beat egg yolks until pale yellow. Slowly add milk mixture to egg yolks, making sure to keep stirring until blended.

2. Whip cream and fold into egg mixture. Add vanilla. Pour into 8 custard cups, and chill before serving.

RECIPE FOR SUCCESS

This recipe gives you great old-fashioned comfort and nourishment. Enhance the creamy texture and taste by garnishing with mint sprigs or berries—or simply use nothing at all.

Slow Cooker Chocolate-Amaretto Cheesecake

Yield:	Serving size:	Prep time:	Cook time:
12 servings	$\frac{1}{12}$ recipe	15 minutes plus 1 to 2 hours standing time and overnight chilling	$2\frac{1}{2}$ to 3 hours

Each serving has:		
16 g carbohydrate	1 g fiber	6 g protein

1 cup ricotta cheese	$\frac{1}{4}$ cup amaretto liqueur
12 oz. cream cheese ($1\frac{1}{2}$ (8-oz.) packages)	$\frac{1}{4}$ cup plus 1 TB. unsweetened cocoa powder
$\frac{1}{2}$ cup sugar	$\frac{1}{4}$ cup flour
2 large eggs	1 tsp. vanilla extract
3 TB. whipping cream	$\frac{1}{3}$ cup semisweet chocolate chips

1. Beat ricotta cheese and cream cheese with sugar until smooth; add eggs and whipping cream, and beat with a handheld electric mixer on medium for about 3 minutes. Add amaretto, cocoa powder, flour, and vanilla; beat for about 1 more minute. Stir in chocolate chips, and pour mixture into a 7-inch springform pan.

2. Place a cheesecake pan on a rack in a slow cooker (or use a "ring" of aluminum foil to keep it off the bottom of the cooker). Cover and cook on high for $2\frac{1}{2}$ to 3 hours. Let stand in the covered cooker (after turning it off) for about 1 to 2 hours, until cool enough to handle. Cool thoroughly before removing sides of pan. Chill before serving, and store leftovers in the refrigerator.

3. Because of the time involved in cooling and chilling, this dessert is best made the day before serving.

RECIPE FOR SUCCESS

This cheesecake is high in complete protein and low in carbs, plus it blends two wonderful flavors into a luscious dessert. By using the slow cooker, the cheesecake comes out very moist.

TABLE TALK

To lower the carbohydrate count of other cheesecake recipes, eliminate the crust. Make the recipe as normal, with the same size pan and same bake time.

Chocolate Truffles

Yield:	**Serving size:**	**Prep time:**	**Cook time:**
24 servings	1 truffle	20 minutes plus chill time	10 minutes

Each serving has:		
5 g carbohydrate	0 g fiber	0 g protein

¼ cup heavy cream	4 TB. butter, at room temperature
2 TB. Grand Marnier	Unsweetened cocoa powder
6 oz. semisweet chocolate chips	

1. Carefully heat cream in a small pan until warm. Remove from heat, and stir in Grand Marnier and chocolate chips. Stir until chocolate melts.

2. Stir in butter, 1 tablespoon at a time, until well blended. Pour into a shallow bowl, and refrigerate until firm.

3. Shape chocolate mixture into 24 (1-inch) balls, and roll balls in unsweetened cocoa. Store in the refrigerator. Bring to room temperature to serve.

RECIPE FOR SUCCESS

You definitely can enjoy the wonderful luscious taste of divinely rich chocolate for only 5 grams carbohydrate. But savor it slowly; make it last. Substitute another liqueur for the Grand Marnier, or leave it out entirely and use water.

Yes, these are actually candy. Yes, there is such a thing as low-carb candy made with real ingredients. One piece goes a long way toward satisfying your sweet tooth, or chocolate tooth, as the case may be.

Nut Clusters

Yield:	Serving size:	Prep time:	Cook time:
24 servings	1 nut cluster	15 minutes plus standing time	None

Each serving has:		
11 g carbohydrate	2 g fiber	1 g protein

2 cups (12-oz.) semisweet chocolate morsels

1 cup pecans

½ cup flaked or shredded coconut, unsweetened

1. Melt chocolate morsels in a microwave or in the top of a double boiler over boiling water. Stir until smooth. Add pecans and coconut, and stir until well blended.

2. Drop by teaspoonfuls onto waxed paper or aluminum foil. Cool.

Variation: Instead of pecans, substitute other nuts, such as peanuts, cashews, walnuts, pine nuts, or pistachios. You can omit the coconut, and add ½ cup more nuts.

Walnut Cake with Chocolate Cream

Yield:	Serving size:	Prep time:	Cook time:
16 servings	1/16 recipe	30 minutes plus chill time	25 to 30 minutes

Each serving has:		
13 g carbohydrate	2 g fiber	7 g protein

10 oz. English walnuts

6 large eggs, separated

¾ cup sugar

½ cup unsweetened chocolate

3 TB. sugar

1½ cups heavy cream

1. Preheat the oven to 350°F.

2. Butter and flour 2 (9-inch) cake pans. Process walnuts in a food processor or a blender until they become a fine powder.

3. In a large bowl, beat egg whites until stiff. In a separate bowl, beat egg yolks until pale yellow and fluffy. Gradually beat sugar into egg yolks, and fold mixture into egg whites. Fold in powdered walnuts.

4. Pour batter into the cake pans, and bake 25 to 30 minutes or until cake is lightly browned. Remove from the oven, and immediately invert the pans on racks. Cool slightly, remove cakes from the pans, and cool thoroughly while preparing Chocolate Cream.

5. Over medium heat, melt chocolate. Stir in sugar, then cream. Stir until mixture almost boils and then remove from heat and chill.

6. When ready to frost cake, beat Chocolate Cream until it's the consistency of whipped cream. Spread Chocolate Cream between layers, on top, and on sides of cake.

RECIPE FOR SUCCESS

This is a fancy cake for special times and celebrations. Your guests will be amazed that this is low carb. You can substitute hazelnuts for the walnuts if you wish.

Chocolate Ganache

Yield:	Serving size:	Prep time:	Cook time:
48 servings	1 tablespoon	5 minutes plus chill time	10 minutes

Each serving has:		
4 g carbohydrate	0 g fiber	0 g protein

1 cup heavy cream

11 oz. semisweet chocolate chips

1 TB. Grand Marnier

1. In a saucepan, scald cream by heating to just below boiling, when small bubbles form around the edges.

2. Remove from heat, and gently stir in chocolate until smooth and melted. Stir in Grand Marnier. Cool and serve over ice cream, brownies, and other desserts. Yields 3 cups.

Rich Chocolate Brownies

Yield: 16 servings	Serving size: 1 brownie or $^1/_{16}$ recipe	Prep time: 20 minutes	Cook time: 30 to 35 minutes
Each serving has: 19 g carbohydrate	2 g fiber	3 g protein	

$1^1/_2$ cups semisweet chocolate

$1^1/_2$ cups milk chocolate

$^3/_4$ cup butter

$^2/_3$ cup ground pecans

3 extra large eggs, slightly beaten

1. Preheat the oven to 350°F.

2. Line the base and sides of an 8-inch-square cake pan with baking parchment or waxed paper.

3. Break semisweet chocolate and $^1/_4$ milk chocolate into pieces, and put into the top of a double boiler. Add butter. Melt over simmering water, stirring frequently. Remove from heat. Stir ground pecans and eggs into melted chocolate.

4. Chop remaining $1^1/_4$ cups milk chocolate into chunky pieces. Stir half of remaining chopped milk chocolate into the warm mixture, and pour into the prepared pan, spreading it into the corners. Milk chocolate doesn't need to melt all the way. Sprinkle with remaining $^1/_2$ cup plus 1 tablespoon chopped milk chocolate.

5. Bake brownies for 30 to 35 minutes, until they rise and are just firm to the touch. Let cool in the pan and then cut into 16 squares.

RECIPE FOR SUCCESS

These are very chocolaty, very rich, and definitely satisfying. You can serve garnished with strawberries or raspberries to keep the carb count low. Or you can serve with a spoonful of ice cream, but remember to count the carbs in the ice cream as part of your daily allotment.

Chocolate Drop Cookies

Yield:	Serving size:	Prep time:	Cook time:
20 servings	1 cookie	10 minutes	20 minutes

Each serving has:			
6 g carbohydrate	1 g fiber	2 g protein	

½ cup butter (1 stick)

½ cup sugar

1 tsp. molasses

1 egg

¼ cup unsweetened cocoa powder

½ tsp. vanilla extract

½ tsp. salt

1¾ cups almond flour (1½ cups almonds, finely ground)

1. Preheat the oven to 300°F.

2. Cream butter with sugar and molasses. Beat in egg. Add cocoa powder, vanilla, and salt. Gradually add almond flour, and mix to a stiff dough. Form into 20 balls, and place balls on a greased cookie sheet about 1 inch apart. Flatten slightly. Bake for 20 minutes.

Variation: You can add ¼ cup unsweetened coconut to the batter or even ½ cup chocolate chips. These variations will increase the carb count.

RECIPE FOR SUCCESS

Sometimes a chocolate cookie hits the spot. And low carbs make it better. These are richer than a normal cookie. You can frost with a teaspoon of Chocolate Ganache (see recipe earlier in this chapter) on top, but it will increase the carb count. Just make sure the cookies have cooled before frosting them.

The Least You Need to Know

- Chocolate is actually good for you.
- This "food fit for the gods" can be an enjoyable part of low-carb eating.
- Use the best-quality ingredients you can find, being sure to use full-fat dairy products in these recipes.
- Eat half a serving to get fewer carbs and still enjoy the taste of chocolate.

Glycemic Index and Carbohydrate List

The following table lists the glycemic index ranking and the carbohydrate content of the ingredients used in the recipes in this book.

Food	Glycemic Index Value	Amount	Carbs (g)	Fiber (g)	Nutritive Carbs
Almond flour	0	1 cup	21	11	10
Almonds	0	1 cup	28	15	13
Apple	38	1 medium	22	5	17
Apple juice	40	1 cup	25	0	25
Apricots	57	3 medium	11	1	10
Apricots, dried	30	1/4 cup	25	2	23
Avocado, California	0	1 medium	12	9	3
Banana	52	1 medium	29	4	25
Barley, pearl, uncooked	25	1/4 cup	37	6	31
Basmati rice, uncooked	58	1/4 cup	33	2	31
Beef	0	any amount	0	0	0
Black beans, boiled	30	1/2 cup	20	8	12
Black-eyed peas, canned	42	1/2 cup	16	4	12
Brazil nut	0	6 large	4	2	2
Broccoli, raw, chopped	0	1/2 cup	2	1	1
Cabbage, raw, shredded	0	1/2 cup	2	1	1

continued

Food	Glycemic Index Value	Amount	Carbs (g)	Fiber (g)	Nutritive Carbs
Cantaloupe, cubed	65	1 cup	13	2	11
Capers	0	1 TB.	1	0	1
Carrots, raw, shredded	47	½ cup	6	2	4
Cashews	22	¼ cup	8	3	5
Cauliflower, 1-inch pieces	0	½ cup	3	2	1
Celery, diced	0	½ cup	2	1	1
Celery root, or celeriac	0	½ cup	7.2	1.4	5.8
Cheese, cheddar and Parmesan	0	1 ounce	0	0	0
Cherries, sweet with pits	22	½ cup	12	2	10
Chickpeas, canned	42	½ cup	18	7	11
Cocoa powder	55	1 TB.	3	1	2
Coconut, shredded, not packed	0	1 cup	12	7	5
Corn, sweet, boiled	60	½ cup	15	5	10
Cornmeal	68	¼ cup	25	3	22
Cornstarch	N/A	1 TB.	9	0	9
Couscous, uncooked	65	¼ cup	35	2	33
Cream, heavy	0	½ cup	3	0	3
Cucumber, sliced	0	½ cup	1.4	0.4	1
Dates	50	¼ cup	32	3	29
Eggs, large	0	1 large	0.6	0	0.6
Fennel, sliced	0	1 cup	6	2	4
Figs, dried	61	¼ cup	26	5	21
Flour	70	¼ cup	22	0	22
Garlic	0	1 clove	1	0.1	0.9
Grapefruit	25	½ medium	16	6	10

Food	Glycemic Index Value	Amount	Carbs (g)	Fiber (g)	Nutritive Carbs
Grapefruit juice	48	1 cup	23	0	23
Grapes, green	46	1½ cups	24	1	23
Green beans, cooked	0	½ cup	5	2	3
Green onions	0	¼ cup	2	1	1
Green peas, frozen	48	⅔ cup	12	4	8
Hazelnuts, diced	0	1 cup	18	7	11
Honey	55	1 TB.	17	0	17
Ice cream, high-fat, vanilla	38	½ cup	16	0	16
Ice cream, low-fat, vanilla	50	½ cup	18	0	18
Jicama	0	½ cup	5	3	2
Kidney beans, boiled	46	½ cup	20	7	13
Kiwi fruit	58	1 medium	11	3	8
Lamb	0	any amount	0	0	0
Leafy vegetables, raw	0	1 cup	2	1	1
Lentils, cooked	29	½ cup	20	8	12
Lima beans, frozen	32	½ cup	22	5	17
Macadamia nuts	0	¼ cup	5	3	2
Mango, sliced	51	1 cup	28	3	25
Milk, full fat	31	1 cup	49	0	49
New potato, boiled	78	½ cup	16	2	14
Oat bran	N/A	½ cup	25	6	19
Oat flour	N/A	⅓ cup	21	3	18
Oatmeal, cooked	42	½ cup	13	2	11
Onion, chopped	0	½ cup	7	1	6
Orange, sections	42	1 cup	19	4	15
Orange juice	53	1 cup	27	0	27
Papaya, sliced	56	1 cup	14	3	11
Peach, sliced	42	1 cup	19	3	16

continues

continued

Food	Glycemic Index Value	Amount	Carbs (g)	Fiber (g)	Nutritive Carbs
Peanuts, roasted	14	¼ cup	12	2	10
Pear	38	1 medium	25	4	21
Pecan flour	0	1 cup	15	15	0
Pecans, half	0	¼ cup	5	5	0
Pepper, red or green, diced	0	¾ cup	4	2	2
Pine nuts	0	¼ cup	5	2	3
Pineapple, diced	66	½ cup	10	1	9
Pinto beans, canned	45	½ cup	18	6	12
Plums, sliced	39	½ cup	11	1	10
Pork	0	any amount	0	0	0
Potato, white, baked in skin	85	4¾ × 2½ inches	51	5	46
Psyllium husks	0	3 TB.	8	8	0
Raisins	64	¼ cup	31	2	29
Rice, brown, uncooked	50	¼ cup	37	3	34
Rice flour	N/A	¼ cup	31	1	30
Salami	0	1 ounce	0	0	0
Shellfish, seafood	0	any amount	0	0	0
Soy flour	N/A	½ cup	16	8	8
Split peas, uncooked	32	¼ cup	27	11	16
Squash, cooked, cubed	0	1 cup	15	2	13
Sucrose, table sugar	68	½ cup	100	0	100
Sweet potato, mashed	44	½ cup	24	3	21
Tomato, chopped	0	1 cup	8	2	6
Tuna and fish	0	any amount	0	0	0
Veal	0	any amount	0	0	0
Vital wheat gluten	N/A	1 TB.	3	0	3

Food	Glycemic Index Value	Amount	Carbs (g)	Fiber (g)	Nutritive Carbs
Walnuts	0	¼ cup	3	3	0
Wild rice, uncooked	57	¼ cup	34	3	31
Wheat germ	N/A	2 TB.	7	4	3
Whey powder	N/A	⅓ cup	2	0	2
Whole-wheat flour	71	¼ cup	21	3	18
Yams, cooked, cubed	37	½ cup	19	3	16

Each ingredient has a glycemic index ranking (GI). This indicates how much your blood sugar level increases when you eat this food. The ranking is based on 100—the lower the number, the less likely the food will trigger a quick rise in blood sugar.

A quick rise in blood sugar stimulates the pancreas to secrete the hormone insulin. Insulin lowers the blood sugar level to a safe range. When the body has a high increase in blood sugar as when eating a high-glycemic food, the pancreas, in a sense, produces more insulin than needed. Excess insulin results in …

* A person getting hungry again soon after eating.

* Increased body-fat storage.

* Increased overall inflammation levels.

* Increased risk of chronic health conditions such as autoimmune disorders, high blood pressure, heart disease, arthritis, and cancer.

Because you don't want these things to happen in your body, it's best to eat low- to moderate-GI foods.

High	> 70
Medium	56 to 69
Low	< 55

The only ingredients we use in this cookbook that are high GI are white potatoes and wheat flour. However, we have used them in such small quantities that their overall effect is minimal.

Listed with the GI of each ingredient is the carbohydrate count based on the amount of food. Use this information to figure the carbohydrate count of other recipes and foods you might eat.

Index

C

G

H

I-J-K

L

N